PEACE,

LOVE

&

FIBRE

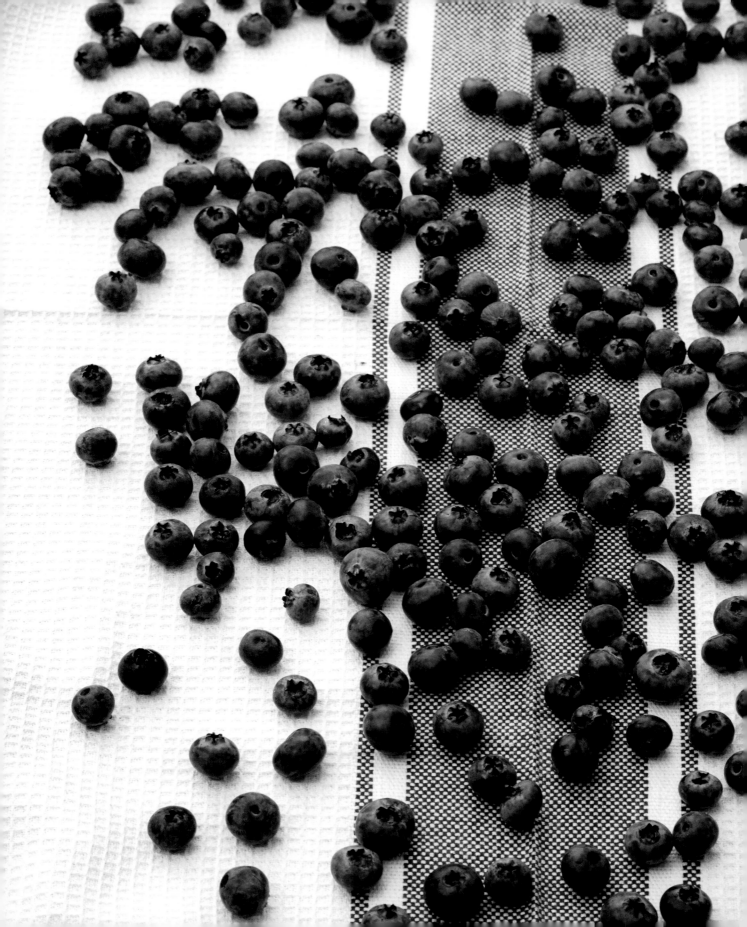

PEACE,

LOVE

&

FIBRE

Over 100 Fibre-Rich Recipes for the Whole Family

Mairlyn Smith, PHEc.

appetite
by RANDOM HOUSE

Appetite by Random House® and colophon are registered trademarks of Penguin Random House LLC.

Library and Archives of Canada Cataloguing in Publication is available upon request.

ISBN: 978-0-14-753092-9
eBook ISBN: 978-0-14-753093-6

Cover and book design by Lisa Jager
Photography by Mike McColl
Food styling by Joan Ttooulias
Chart on page 4 by the Dietitians of Canada
(http://www.unlockfood.ca/en/Articles/
Fibre/Focus-on-Fibre.aspx)

Printed and bound in China

Published in Canada by Appetite by Random House®, a division of Penguin Random House LLC.

www.penguinrandomhouse.ca

10 9 8 7 6 5 4 3 2 1

appetite
by RANDOM HOUSE | Penguin
Random House
Canada

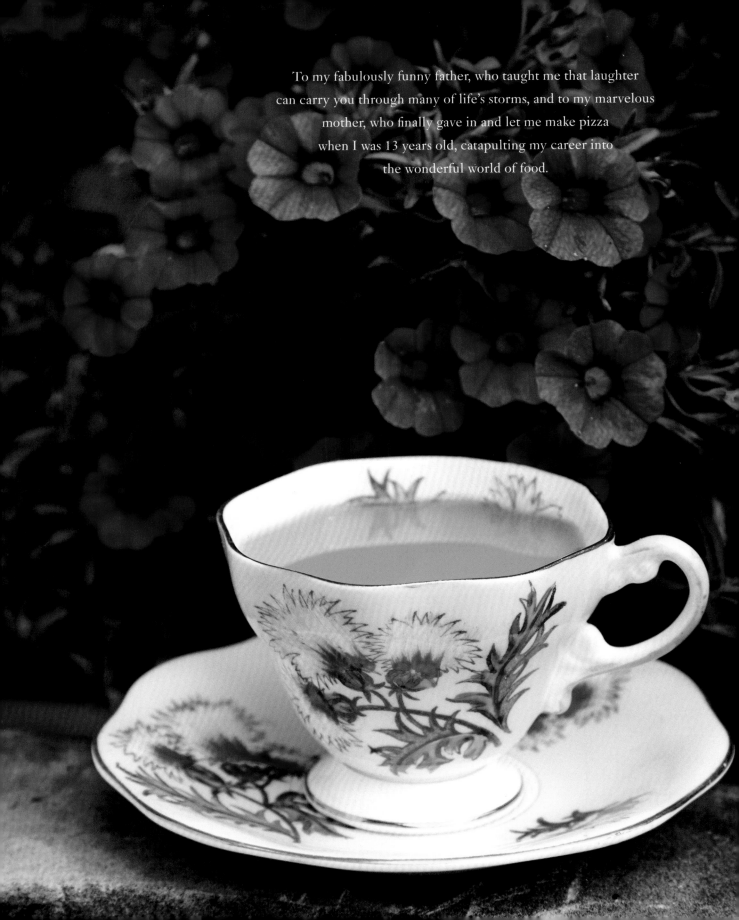

To my fabulously funny father, who taught me that laughter can carry you through many of life's storms, and to my marvelous mother, who finally gave in and let me make pizza when I was 13 years old, catapulting my career into the wonderful world of food.

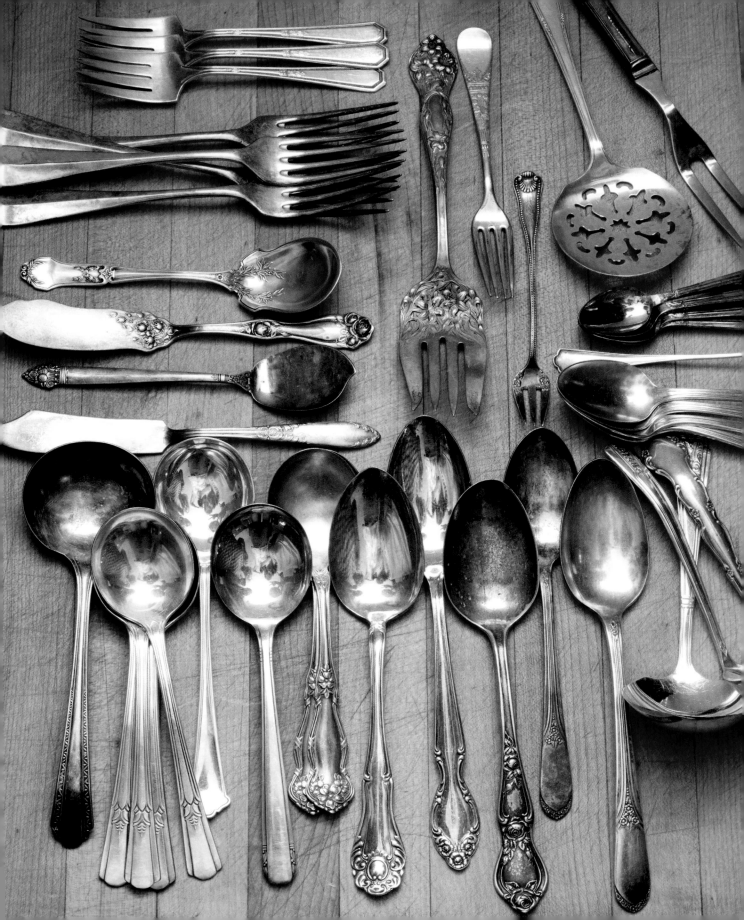

CONTENTS

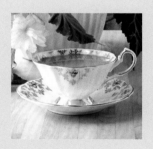

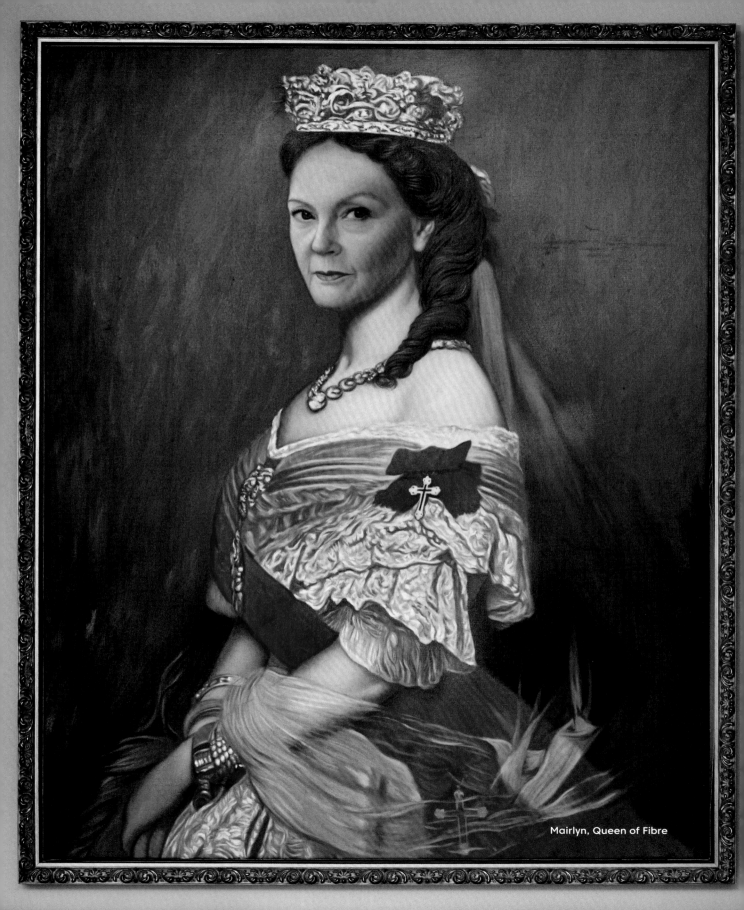

Mairlyn, Queen of Fibre

Introduction

A HEALTHY LIFESTYLE IS ABOUT MORE THAN just what you eat. It's about how you cope with stress, how much you exercise, your social circles, your faith, how you face adversity, and a myriad of other factors.

If you eat 10 servings of vegetables and fruit every day but aren't getting enough sleep, are eating highly processed foods regularly, are playing on your devices, and then are becoming an inert couch potato from 7 p.m. until bedtime, your long-term health can easily become affected in a negative way. Those vegetables and fruits are only part of what we call a healthy lifestyle.

To live your optimal life, you need to nurture not only your body, but your spirit as well—I always remind myself that health is not the absence of illness, but the total package of my life's choices. It's because of my belief in the power of mind, body, and spirit working all together that my sign-off is to wish everyone peace, love, and fibre. But talk is cheap. I know you're wondering how I put these three ideas together to create my own healthy lifestyle.

I find peace in the quiet moments I spend each day being thankful for the life that I have, and in drinking tea out of my good teacups. I find peace whenever I reach out to others and offer help and kindness. Or when my husband and I go for a ride in the country, listening to music and walking in nature. I get love from my family and friends, and from loving what I do for a living: writing cookbooks and encouraging people to take care of themselves and their bodies. And fibre? Well, fibre and I go way back. I believe that without fibre in your diet, you'll never be on top of your game—either physically or mentally.

My faith in fibre started when I was studying foods and nutrition at the University of British Columbia, and it has grown exponentially over the years. As the health benefits of fibre kept popping up in my life, they spurred me on to create fibre-rich recipes.

My passion for the power of fibre escalated when I read an Australian study published in 2016 that indicated that a diet high in fibre was a key predictor of what the researchers called "successful aging." They found that people who ate a diet rich in fibre had an almost 80% greater likelihood of living a long and healthy life. Those high-fibre eaters were also less likely to suffer from disability, depression, dementia, respiratory problems, heart disease, stroke, and cancer. Yes, the big C-word. Eating fibre had long been linked to a reduction in heart disease and type 2 diabetes, but cancer? That really got my attention.

That same year, findings from the Nurses' Health Study II showed that women eating a high-fibre diet reduced their chances of developing breast cancer. The earlier they adopted a high-fibre eating lifestyle, the better the protection.

All this exciting news about fibre's positive effects on heart disease, type 2 diabetes, depression, dementia, and cancer is worthy of a 21-gun salute, yet fibre just doesn't get the respect it deserves.

My mission is to change that.

As the self-appointed Queen of Fibre, I want you to start adding more fibre to your day, every day. No matter what your eating style is, I'm here to help make that happen, one tip, one ingredient, one recipe at a time.

Incorporate fibre into your eating style and embrace the power of peace and love.

Wishing you all
peace, love, and fibre—

Fibre 101 or How to Get an A+ on Your Colonoscopy

"EAT MORE FIBRE." YOU'VE HEARD THIS BEFORE and you're going to hear it in the future, because fibre is exceptionally good for your short-term and long-term health.

But why? What *is* the big deal about fibre anyway?

To understand the why, you first must know the what.

What Is Fibre & What Does It Do?

I could wow you with a long, amazing dissertation on this topic, but here's the mini version: fibre is a type of carbohydrate that the body can't truly digest. Fibre can't be broken down into sugar molecules like most other carbohydrates can, so it passes through the body undigested. And that's a very good thing. These undigested carbohydrates help keep your blood sugar levels on an even keel instead of ricocheting around like a crazed pinball machine. This is a tremendous plus for anyone living with diabetes, but also for anyone in general.

There are two main types of fibre, insoluble and soluble, and both are extremely important. Insoluble fibre does not absorb water; its main function is to keep everything moving through your gastrointestinal (GI) tract. Eating enough insoluble fibre will help prevent constipation and keep you regular. Some great sources of insoluble fibre are whole grains, most vegetables, wheat bran, and nuts.

Soluble fibre does absorb water, and its main function is to help lower your blood sugar levels and your blood cholesterol. Because it dissolves in water and becomes a viscous goo, it makes you feel fuller longer and gives you a softer, albeit bulkier, stool. It sounds gross, I know, but it's important to understand. Some great sources of soluble fibre are all beans, especially black and kidney beans, oats, barley, flaxseed, Brussels sprouts, broccoli, sweet potato, eggplant, avocado, orange, pear, apricot, apple, and psyllium (found in Metamucil).

Probiotics & Prebiotics

I can't talk about fibre and gut health without mentioning probiotics and prebiotics. As many of you know, we have both good and bad bacteria in our bodies, but we need to make sure that we have more good than bad. Probiotics are living microorganisms, and prebiotics are integral to their function.

Probiotics, or the good guys, as I like to call them, contribute to the ecosystem of the gut by creating a physical barrier against the bad bacteria. They can also improve the health of your digestive tract and its ability to absorb nutrients. Ongoing research suggests that probiotics can help people suffering from diarrhea due to antibiotic use, living with Crohn's disease or colitis, or experiencing irritable bowel syndrome, H. Pylori (a bacteria infection that may cause certain types of ulcers), urinary tract infections, or vaginal infections.

Researchers are even looking at probiotics and their effects on such diverse health issues as depression, acne, autism, gut cell-wall health in HIV-1-positive patients, and colon cancer. It's too early in the research chain to give ringing endorsements, but the fact that scientists are looking at links is exciting to me.

PROBIOTICS ARE FOUND IN THE FOLLOWING FERMENTED AND CULTURED PRODUCTS:

- Miso—fermented soybean paste used in Japanese cuisine, mostly for soup
- Kombucha—fermented tea
- Tempeh—a soy product
- Kimchi—fermented pickled cabbage
- Sauerkraut—fermented cabbage
- Fermented pickles

- Olives in brine
- Buttermilk
- Yogurt—look for "live cultures" or "active cultures" in the ingredient list
- Kefir—look for "live cultures" in the ingredient list

The bottom line for me is this: eat probiotic-rich foods daily. But be careful not to overdo it. You can eat too many good-for-you foods in just the same way as you can eat too many bad-for-you foods. Moderation is key. I eat either yogurt or kefir every day, but my intake of the other foods on this list is more occasional.

Prebiotics are non-digestible carbohydrates found in certain fibre foods that act as food for the gut bacteria. They support the good guys in gut health. Some of my favourite sources of prebiotics are whole grains, especially oats and barley, and the entire family in the Wonderful World of Pulses: beans, split peas, lentils, and chickpeas. You'll also find prebiotics in bananas, onions, garlic, asparagus, and artichokes.

Fermentation: The New Kid on the Fibre Block

Certain fibres ferment in the large intestine. Fermenting in the gut? That can't be good, right? Wrong! Because your body can't digest fibre, the bacteria in your gut kick in and digest it for you, producing the energy for the cells that line your colon, which is extremely important for your colon health and overall immunity. The two biggest stars of fermentable fibre appear to be barley and oats, which I use throughout this cookbook.

✳

WHAT ABOUT FIBRE-FORTIFIED FOODS? EATING FIBRE-FORTIFIED FOODS CAN INCREASE YOUR OVERALL FIBRE INTAKE, BUT THE FOODS THAT ARE FORTIFIED TEND NOT TO BE THE BEST BANG FOR YOUR NUTRITIONAL BUCK. A BETTER CHOICE IS TO EAT FIBRE-RICH FOODS.

✳

Resistant Starch

Resistant starch is a form of starch found in foods such as cold cooked potatoes, underripe bananas, pulses (beans, split peas, lentils, and chickpeas), cold cooked rice, and seeds that can't be digested. They perform just like a prebiotic. It's a win-win for gut health, which in turn is a win-win for your general health. There's just a whole lot of winning going on when it comes to eating fibre-rich foods.

Can Fibre Help You Lose Weight?

Soluble fibre fills you up because of that viscous goo I mentioned earlier. When you feel full after eating a food rich in soluble fibre, like a bowl of steel-cut oats first thing in the morning, it's because your body is processing that fibre, which bulks up in your gut and helps reduce circulating blood sugars. Feeling full may help you lose weight because your appetite decreases and you eat fewer calories.

According to a study published in 2014, if fibre is as good for humans as it is for male rats, then the answer is yes, you will lose weight. This is also why certain companies that produce products to aid in constipation are also touting their products as weight-loss aids. Psyllium, used in one such product, is a soluble fibre, which helps with constipation as well as satiety.

Colorectal Cancer

In 2017, according to the Canadian Cancer Society, colorectal cancer was the second-most common cancer diagnosed in Canada, the second-leading cause of death from cancer in men, and the third-leading cause of death from cancer in women.

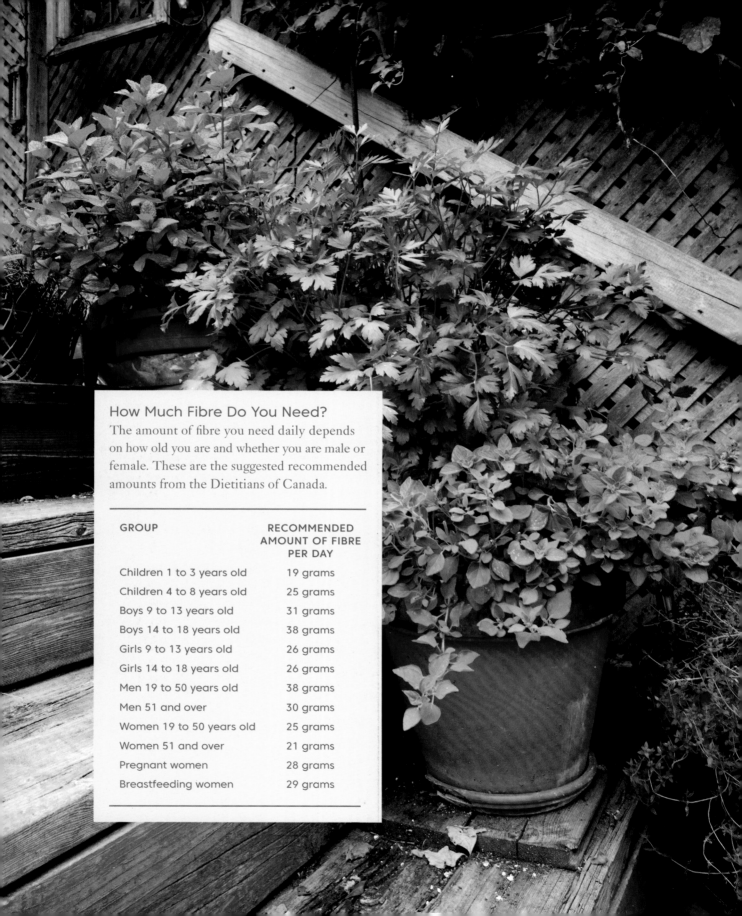

How Much Fibre Do You Need?

The amount of fibre you need daily depends on how old you are and whether you are male or female. These are the suggested recommended amounts from the Dietitians of Canada.

GROUP	RECOMMENDED AMOUNT OF FIBRE PER DAY
Children 1 to 3 years old	19 grams
Children 4 to 8 years old	25 grams
Boys 9 to 13 years old	31 grams
Boys 14 to 18 years old	38 grams
Girls 9 to 13 years old	26 grams
Girls 14 to 18 years old	26 grams
Men 19 to 50 years old	38 grams
Men 51 and over	30 grams
Women 19 to 50 years old	25 grams
Women 51 and over	21 grams
Pregnant women	28 grams
Breastfeeding women	29 grams

In the United States, according to the American Cancer Society, colorectal cancer is the third-most common cancer diagnosed in both men and women and the third-leading cause of cancer-related deaths in both men and women.

Currently in Canada, the baseline age for a colonoscopy is 50 years old, unless you have a predisposition. If you have a family member who has had colon cancer or polyps, or if you're African-American, you should be screened sooner. Talk to your doctor about it.

Years ago, one of my comedy buddies in my touring company at Second City was diagnosed with colon cancer. After he was finished treatment, a wild and crazy party was organized to celebrate. He spoke that night about the power of the colonoscopy and early detection and urged us to take part in a large study on colon cancer being held in Toronto. I wanted to be a part of the bigger picture and help science, so I immediately signed up.

Weeks later I was interviewed to become a volunteer in the study. I was so nervous—I mean, what if I didn't pass? How pathetic would that be? What if the self-proclaimed Queen of Fibre got rejected for a study on poop, bowel function, and GI health? That would be an insult to my belief in the power of fibre.

Fortunately, or so I thought, I passed that test and was given a poop bucket to take home with me. The subway was really crowded that day; I had to stand holding the bar and a yellow poop bucket labelled "Hazardous Waste." I knew people were staring, but I proudly clutched that bucket all the way home. I was helping science! I felt incredibly virtuous. The deal was, you pooped

*

"POPULATIONS THAT CONSUME MORE DIETARY FIBRE HAVE LESS CHRONIC DISEASE. IN ADDITION, INTAKE OF DIETARY FIBRE HAS BENEFICIAL EFFECTS ON RISK FACTORS FOR DEVELOPING SEVERAL CHRONIC DISEASES."

*

*Academy of Nutrition
and Dietetics*

into the bucket and called a hotline, and a poop collector would come to your house within a specific time to ensure the poop was fresh, then rush it back to the lab.

Weeks later, after my colonoscopy prep (one of the most explosive preps known to man—enough said!), I showed up at the hospital only to be told that I had arrived one week early. Despite my begging, cajoling, crying, guilt-tripping ("I'm participating in a colon cancer study for the betterment of mankind!"), and, in one of the lowest-of-the-low moments of my life, throwing down the "I'm on TV" card, the receptionist was a rock and wouldn't budge.

I was instructed to come back in several months so I could go through the whole shebang again. I quietly left the building, hat in hand, and did not submit myself to another colonoscopy prep until I was 50. Fortunately, this time I got the date right, had the colonoscopy, and received an A+. The doctor told me I had the most beautiful colon he'd ever seen, and apparently, he'd seen a million of them—he seemed close to 100 years old. I've considered having this carved on my tombstone:

*Here lies Mairlyn Smith:
She had the most beautiful
colon ever seen.*
Signed, *The Unknown
Centenarian Colon Doctor*

You too can get an A+ on your colonoscopy by eating healthy, back-to-basic foods that include fibre-rich vegetables and fruits, berries, whole grains, nuts, seeds, pulses, and fermented foods, as well as going for a walk every day and drinking enough liquids to keep your GI tract happy and moving. It's never too late to start adding fibre-rich foods to your diet. This is the main reason I decided to write this cookbook. Although eating a lifetime of high-fibre foods is great, adding them to your eating style as of today is the best news your body will have heard in ages. Think of it as an investment in your retirement health savings plan. The sooner you start adding to it, the better. Your body is going to be on the winning end, pun intended.

Easy Does It

You've been reading "Fibre 101 or How to Get an A+ on Your Colonoscopy," and now you're ready to jump on the fibre bandwagon. Excellent! Insert an image of me doing a happy dance. But before you go all fibre-crazy, bear in mind that too much too soon could be a recipe for gastrointestinal disaster.

Even though fibre is good for you, an increase in your fibre intake needs to be gradual or you could experience bloating, abdominal pain, gas, and diarrhea. No one wants to sign up for that. Give your digestive system time to make friends with fibre. Depending on how low your fibre intake was before you bought this cookbook, it can take months before you're eating the recommended amount for your age and gender (see page 4).

If you're like the majority of the population, you're probably getting only half of the recommended daily intake of fibre, somewhere in the ballpark of 12 to 16 grams per day. Doubling your fibre in the first day is plain crazy. Your digestive tract will not be pleased, and you might even miss a day of work.

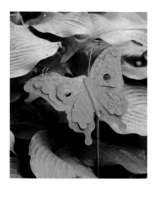

Start by adding a small amount of extra fibre in two-week increments. For two weeks, add 4 to 6 grams of fibre to your daily intake than you were previously consuming—this is the equivalent of adding a large apple or sprinkling 1 tablespoon of ground flaxseed onto your morning cereal or yogurt and adding half a banana. For the next two weeks, add another 4 to 6 grams to your daily intake, until you and your body are at the recommended level and you're feeling fabulous and having great bowel movements (BMs).

Don't Forget the Water

Fibre needs liquids.

Fibre loves absorbing liquids and then travelling on its merry way through your digestive system. You're aiming for a balance between fibre and liquids so you're having easy, soft BMs. Too little liquid plus too much fibre results in hard BMs—basically the recipe for cement poop in your bowel. The reverse is true as well: fibre and too much liquid can result in diarrhea.

Most days I eat at least 25 to 30 grams of fibre and drink about six glasses (that's a 1-cup measure) of liquids, mostly water, and I have lovely BMs. But that's my body. Yours could be very different. Let your body be your guide. This isn't about being on a fad diet or in a race to better health; it's a forever-healthy style of eating. You're better off to go slowly and find out what works best for you.

Now let's talk about the elephant in the room. Warning: the following may offend anyone who doesn't like thinking about farting, never mind reading about it. But the fact is, we all fart. On average, we break wind 14 times a day. And that's normal. And yes, fibre can make you rip one more often until your body gets used to the extra roughage.

Here's the thing: our digestive

tract or gastrointestinal (GI) tract is an extraordinary piece of mechanical engineering. It's extremely busy breaking down your food into proteins, fats, carbohydrates, vitamins, and minerals. When broken down, some foods produce more toots than other foods. That gas must exit your body somehow, be it a burp or a fit of flatulence. Sometimes cutting the cheese isn't all that stinky and sometimes you just never know. Hence lies the dilemma: to fart or not to fart?

When I was in my 20s, 30s, and 40s, I never fluffed around anyone. I never let one go anywhere but in the safety of my own home, and if possible, alone. I would rather have imploded than toot in front of another person.

But something happened right around my 50th birthday.

We had just had one of our regular weeknight chili dinners, and my husband, my son, and our dog, Bailey, were all in the family room watching TV when Bailey let off an enormous ripper. (Important to note: Bailey did not eat any of the chili. She just had smelly gas, often.) We all giggled and gagged, and then my son and my husband cut the cheese in unison, and we were all laughing so much I thought, why not join in? I pointed my finger in the universal hand gesture for shooting a gun and let one go. And I'm telling you, it was one of those Oprah Winfrey aha moments. Why had I been cramping up all those years when, in fact, farting openly was liberating and funny? It was one of the most freeing moments of my adult life.

Flatulence is a natural thing, and in some countries it's totally acceptable after an exceptionally good dinner. But in North America,

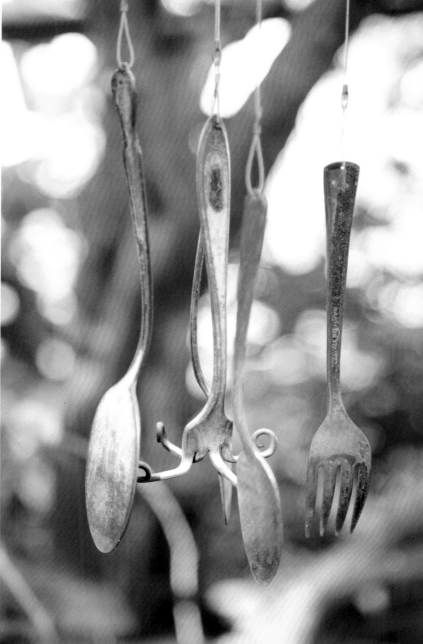

bodily functions are not welcomed in public spaces, especially elevators. I draw the line at openly farting in public, unless there is a completely annoying person standing behind me, in which case, the gloves are off. But in the privacy of my own home, hey, holding them in is silly and not great for my health. I just point and shoot.

Peace, Love & Fibre the Inclusive Way

WHEN I FIRST BECAME A VEGETARIAN, I can't tell you how many times I was invited to someone's house for dinner and served a bowl of peas while everyone else ate a roast beef dinner complete with gravy and Yorkshire puddings cooked in beef drippings. It didn't really bother me, but once I had my own place, I wanted to be an inclusive host as well as an inclusive recipe developer.

I'm no longer a vegetarian, but when company comes over I always ask if they have a food allergy or if they're vegetarian or vegan. Then I make something that everyone will enjoy.

The same thinking applies when someone comes over who is living with celiac disease or is gluten-sensitive. I always have a meal, including a dessert, that will please all my guests. That doesn't mean making one dish for most guests and a special gluten-free dish for the minority; rather, it's about being inclusive throughout.

I created this cookbook to be user-friendly no matter your eating style. There are vegetarian, vegan, lactose-free, and gluten-free recipes, as well as recipes that use gluten, dairy products, meat, pork, and poultry.

THESE SYMBOLS INDICATE A PARTICULAR EATING STYLE:

> Vegetarian = VEG
> Vegan = V
> Lactose Free = LF
> Gluten Free = GF

Nutrient Breakdowns & Carbohydrate Choices

I believe that knowledge is power, so I've included nutrient breakdowns for the recipes. You will be able to see how many grams of fibre a recipe has, as well as how many calories and how many grams of fat, cholesterol, sodium, carbohydrate, sugar, added sugar, protein, and potassium. If you're living with diabetes, I have included the carbohydrate choices to make this cookbook easy and accessible for planning out your meals and snacks. Katie Brunke RD calculated all the nutrient breakdowns and carbohydrate choices in the cookbook.

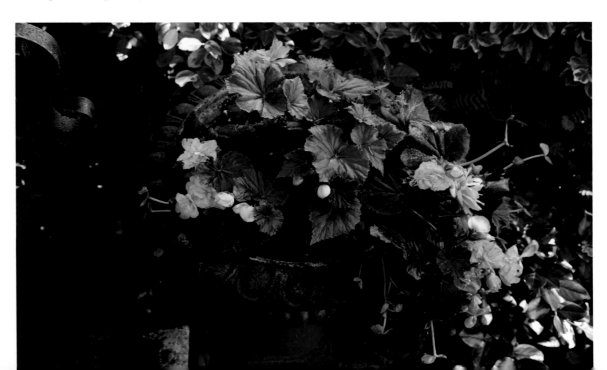

The Peace, Love & High-Fibre Pantry

CHECKING OUT A PANTRY IS LIKE SHINING A light into the soul of the cook. Shine a light into my pantry and you'll see a person who loves to bake from scratch; a person who loves back-to-basics foods such as pulses, nuts, and whole grains; a person who loves fibre; and a person who is a card-carrying chocoholic. Basically, my pantry is an eclectic mix of ingredients from around the world and a whole lotta chocolate.

My pantry is also my best friend in the kitchen. It can save me from a busy-day meltdown by letting me make a quick and easy dinner that's on the table in 20 minutes. It can offer appetizers and snacks if unexpected company drops by, and it can help me whip up a quick batch of brownies when I'm having a "must eat chocolate" moment.

I'm assuming that you all have the basics—you know, baking powder, onions, sweet potatoes, and the usual home pantry items. The most important part about a good pantry is that it contains the ingredients you use most often. If you prefer a different root vegetable to sweet potatoes, I trust that you'll choose that instead. Below are my high-fibre pantry additions to round out your list, along with a few other key ingredients that require additional explanation.

FLOURS

If you haven't gone through these in two months, store whole grain flours in your fridge or freezer or buy in smaller amounts at a bulk food store.

- ☐ Whole grain barley flour
- ☐ Whole grain oat flour
- ☐ Whole grain spelt flour
- ☐ Whole wheat flour
- ☐ Chickpea flour

BAKING BASICS

Be sure to check out my specific High-Fibre Baking Pantry in the Treats chapter on page 184.

- ☐ Dark chocolate (at least 72% cocoa mass)
- ☐ Dark chocolate chips
- ☐ Natural cocoa powder
- ☐ Oat bran
- ☐ Oat flakes, large
- ☐ Steel-cut oats
- ☐ Wheat bran

NUTS AND SEEDS

If you haven't eaten these within three months, store them in your fridge or freezer to increase their shelf life.

- ☐ Natural almond butter or peanut butter
- ☐ Raw almonds
- ☐ Raw cashews
- ☐ Raw pecans
- ☐ Raw pumpkin seeds
- ☐ Raw walnuts
- ☐ Sesame seeds
- ☐ Whole and ground flaxseed

PULSES AND GRAINS

Keep these stored in a cool, dark place.

- ☐ Whole green lentils
- ☐ Split red lentils
- ☐ Split yellow peas
- ☐ Grains (see more about grains on page 13)
- ☐ Pot barley
- ☐ Wheat berries
- ☐ Farro
- ☐ Spelt
- ☐ Quinoa
- ☐ Brown rice

CANNED GOODS

Rotate canned goods regularly.

- ☐ Black beans
- ☐ Chickpeas
- ☐ Mixed beans
- ☐ Red kidney beans
- ☐ White kidney beans
- ☐ Whole green lentils
- ☐ Whole red lentils

FREEZER GOODS

Use within 3 to 6 months.

- ☐ Frozen berries: blueberries, raspberries, strawberries
- ☐ Cornmeal, medium-grind
- ☐ Wheat germ

Some Thoughts on Sugar

Added sugars are often called "free sugars" in the food manufacturing industry and in the world of food science. These sugars are added in the preparation of a food by a food manufacturer, in a recipe, in the kitchen, or at the table. To spot the list of added sugars on a food label, watch for "ose" at the end of a word. Examples are fructose, sucrose, glucose-fructose, dextrose, high-fructose corn syrup, or maltose. Words ending in "ol" like sorbitol and xylitol are types of added sugars as well. Molasses, rice syrup, corn syrup, honey, barley malt, fruit juice concentrate, evaporated cane juice, invert sugar, and maple syrup are also considered added sugars.

Currently, Canadian nutrition labels need to display only the total sugars of a product, which makes it difficult for consumers to differentiate between naturally occurring sugars and the added ones. Consuming too much added sugar has been associated with heart disease, stroke, obesity, diabetes, high blood pressure, and dental cavities.

In 2015 the World Health Organization, concerned about long-term health, set out guidelines for the amount of added or free sugars to be consumed in a day. They recommended that only 10% of a person's total caloric intake, and ideally less than 5%, should come from added sugars or from honey, syrups, or fruit juice.

What does that mean to the consumer? It breaks down to this:

- The average adult female should consume only 6 teaspoons (25 grams) of added sugars a day.
- The average adult male should consume only 9 teaspoons (38 grams) of added sugars a day.

The next time you read a food label, check out the amount of total sugars, and remember that every 4 grams of sugar on the label is equal to 1 teaspoon of sugar—and you won't know if that sugar is naturally occurring or added. On average, North Americans eat 16 to 21 teaspoons of added sugar every day. If it's hard to wrap your head around that number, think twice before you dive into a Venti Vanilla Bean Crème Frappuccino made with whole milk and whipped cream at Starbucks. That weighs in with 18 teaspoons of added sugar. Or consider the iconic Iced Capp at Tim Hortons. A large Iced Capp contains 15 teaspoons of sugar. According to the new guidelines, that's a little more than twice the recommended daily amount for a woman. One mega Slurpee contains 38 teaspoons of sugar, which is a little more than ¾ cup. That's about six times more than the recommendation. And that's just in one soft drink.

The next time you eat an average slice of chocolate cake, keep in mind that there are about 55 grams of total sugars in that one slice—nine times more than is recommended. My recipe for Chocolate Fudge Cake (page 219) has 30.2 grams of total sugars, so it's still a treat, but with a little more than half the sugar of an average piece of chocolate cake.

In this book, I have included the total sugars as well as the added sugars in the nutrient breakdown in every recipe, not just those in the Treats chapter. If you subtract the added sugars from the total sugars, you will see how much sugar is naturally occurring.

✳

WWW.SUGARSCIENCE.ORG IS A WEBSITE FROM A TEAM OF HEALTH SCIENTISTS AT THE UNIVERSITY OF CALIFORNIA, SAN FRANCISCO. THEIR GOAL IS TO HELP CONSUMERS NAVIGATE THROUGH CURRENT SUGAR RESEARCH.

✳

Table Salt

Iodine is an important mineral that our bodies need from food to make thyroid hormones. Adults who don't get enough iodine in their diets can develop a goitre, which is a swelling in the neck, and a low output of thyroid hormone can lead to slower metabolism and poor thinking skills. Table salt contains iodine. One teaspoon of table salt contains 380 micrograms of iodine, which is slightly over the daily recommended amount for adults. The best source of iodine is seafood—as in, saltwater fish. Other high sources are dairy products, whole wheat, red meat, chicken, turkey, and kidney beans.

The sodium added to food products does not contain added iodine. My concern is that if you are eating a restricted diet (eliminating food groups that contain iodine) and eating processed foods or eating out often, you are consuming too much sodium and not enough iodine. Too much sodium may lead to a whole array of cardiac problems. Although kosher salt and sea salt are sources of natural iodine, they may not contain as much as table salt and are not standardized. I eat foods that are good sources of iodine every day, and I use "no-salt-added" products, which helps to reduce the amount of sodium I'm getting in my diet. I add small amounts of table salt to my recipes to get that much-needed iodine, so that's what you'll find in this cookbook.

Oils

My two favourite oils to cook with are extra virgin olive oil and canola oil. I choose authentic Italian extra virgin olive oil, which will have either "DOP" or "IGP" on the label. These seals designate the authenticity of extra virgin olive oil and are your assurance that the olives have been picked and pressed within the designated time, keeping those valuable anti-inflammatory properties in action.

Extra virgin olive oil has a flavour—either grassy, nutty, bitter, or a combo—depending on where the olives were grown. I use extra virgin olive oil in recipes where I want to contribute that flavour to the overall taste of the finished dish as well as to contribute to your heart health. I use canola oil, which has a neutral flavour, when I want to use an oil without a flavour or when there are competing flavours in the dish. Canola oil is heart-healthy and high in valuable omega-3 fatty acids. I also use canola oil for baking, high-heat cooking, marinating, and barbecuing.

La Bomba Antipasto Spread

I add this secret ingredient to Italian cuisine when I want a big hit of spicy, fabulous flavour without much work. It's a finely chopped antipasto-style condiment. I add it to pasta dishes, salad dressings, or dipping sauces. Once opened, it can be stored in your fridge for up to one month.

Garlic

Garlic contains antioxidants, which are great for you, but to ensure that the antioxidants are more bioavailable, you need to oxidize garlic—chop it and let it breathe—before adding it to a recipe. I give it a five- to 20-minute time-out on my counter.

Tamari

Some soy sauces are made with just soybeans, but most soy sauces contain wheat and some may have other ingredients like artificial colours and/or flavourings. Read the label and the list of ingredients. Tamari uses only soybeans and is the by-product of miso paste—and that's it. It's the real deal. It has a richer, deeper flavour than most soy sauces that have added ingredients, so you end up using less. Both soy sauce and tamari are high in sodium, so I choose the lower-sodium version. I use tamari exclusively in the cookbook. Once opened, it can be stored in the fridge for up to two years.

Barley

Barley is the unsung hero in the whole grain world. It is one of the richest sources of both soluble and insoluble fibre. These dietary fibres provide your GI tract with friendly bacteria, which help make it a happy camper—trust me, you don't want 26 feet of angry GI tract. Make nice with your GI tract and it will make nice with you. Barley's true claim to fame lies in its high levels of beta-glucans. This type of soluble fibre helps lower cholesterol and also promotes healthy blood sugar levels by slowing down the absorption of glucose, which is a winning combination for diabetics.

There are two types of barley: pot and pearled. Both have been through a pearling machine, which removes the tough outer hull. Pot barley has gone through the pearling machine for only a short time, keeping some of the bran intact. Pearled barley has gone through the pearling machine for a longer time, removing the bran layer. Regardless of the pearling time, the soluble fibre is still present in either form of barley. Store barley in a cool, dark cupboard or in your fridge for up to one year.

Brown Rice

Rice has higher levels of inorganic arsenic than other foods. Part of it has to do with how and where rice is grown, as well as the fact that rice tends to absorb more arsenic from the soil than other plants. In April 2016, the U.S. Food and Drug Administration (FDA) proposed a limit of arsenic in infant rice cereal and advised a rice consumption level for pregnant women. I limit my consumption to once or twice a week, but that's my personal call. The FDA suggests that rice be cooked with a ratio of 6:1 or 10:1 water to rice and drained after cooking to reduce approximately 50% of the arsenic. Soaking rice overnight can help reduce inorganic arsenic levels further. People following a gluten-free diet, look at your rice options. For many of the gluten-free recipes in the cookbook, I have used either quinoa or brown rice.

Wheat Berries or Hard Wheat Kernels

Wheat berries, or hard wheat kernels, are the real deal when it comes to wheat. They contain the bran, the endosperm, and the germ, making them nutrient-dense. They have a nutty flavour and are fairly chewy, which is one of the reasons I love them.

You can find them in most bulk food stores, sold as either wheat berries, hard wheat kernels, hard red winter wheat, or wheat kernels. Make sure you are buying the full wheat kernels and not a pearled version. The full wheat kernels take around 40 to 60 minutes. I like to cook them with less water than most packages suggest because of the B vitamins these wee kernels offer. B vitamins are water-soluble, so when you cook wheat berries in excess water and drain before serving, you are basically throwing some of the B vitamins down the drain.

Quinoa

There are two common misconceptions about quinoa (pronounced *keen-wah*):

MISCONCEPTION #1: Quinoa is a grain. Wrong. Quinoa is a seed. It cooks like a grain and we eat it as a grain, but it's not a grain.

MISCONCEPTION #2: Quinoa is loaded in protein. Wrong. Quinoa is not very high in protein. It weighs in with 3 grams per ½ cup cooked. It gets its glory from the fact that it's a complete protein, like meat, fish, and poultry, which is hard to find in the plant world.

Grains Cooking Chart

Below are my tried, tested, and true cooking times for the grains used in this cookbook.

BARLEY

1 cup pot barley + 2 cups liquid + 3½-quart saucepan + 35 to 40 minutes = about 3 cups cooked barley

Rinse the barley and let drain. Pour the liquid (water or broth) into a saucepan and add barley. Bring to a boil, cover, and reduce heat to medium-low. There will be bubbling but not a rapid boil. Cook for 35 to 40 minutes. When the water has been absorbed, remove from heat and leave covered for 10 minutes. Fluff with a fork.

LONG-GRAIN BROWN RICE

1 cup long-grain brown rice + 6 cups water + 3½-quart saucepan + 20 to 25 minutes = about 3 cups cooked rice

Soak the rice overnight in 10 cups water for 1 cup rice. Drain and rinse. Pour water into a saucepan and add rice. Bring to a boil, and reduce heat to medium. Cook for 20 to 25 minutes. Remove from heat, drain, return to pot, and cover for 10 minutes. Fluff with a fork.

QUINOA

1 cup quinoa + 2 cups liquid + 3½-quart saucepan + 10 to 14 minutes = about 3 cups cooked quinoa

Rinse the quinoa and let drain. Pour liquid (water or broth) into a saucepan and add quinoa. Bring to a boil, cover, and reduce heat to medium-low. There will be bubbling but not a rapid boil. Cook for 10 to 14 minutes. When the grains are translucent and all of the water has been absorbed, remove from heat and leave covered for 10 minutes. Fluff with a fork.

WHEAT BERRIES

1 cup wheat berries + 2 cups water + 3½-quart saucepan + 35 to 50 minutes = about 2½ cups cooked wheat berries

Rinse the wheat berries and let drain. Add wheat berries and water to a saucepan. Bring to a boil, cover, and reduce heat to medium-low. There will be bubbling but not a rapid boil. Cook for 35 to 50 minutes. Do not let boil dry—check three-quarters of the way through to make sure there is still water in the bottom of the pot. When the water has been absorbed, remove from heat and leave covered for 10 minutes. Fluff with a fork.

Portable Emergency Fibre Snacks

I AM NEVER WITHOUT AN EMERGENCY SNACK
in my purse. Here are my go-to options:

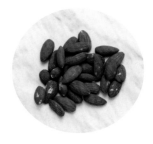

¼ cup almonds:
3.8 grams of fibre

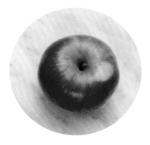

¼ cup walnut halves:
1.7 grams of fibre

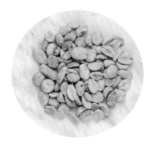

¼ cup peanuts:
3.2 grams of fibre

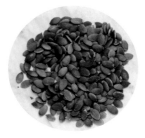

¼ cup raw pumpkin seeds:
1.6 grams of fibre

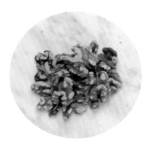

Medium-sized apple:
3.5 grams of fibre

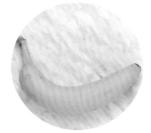

Medium-sized banana:
2.1 grams of fibre

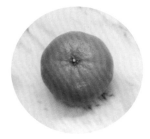

Mandarin orange:
2.3 grams of fibre

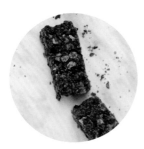

Snack Bar (page 203):
6.3 grams of fibre

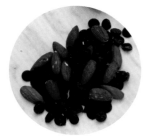

Trail Mix (2 Tbsp chocolate chips
+ 2 Tbsp almonds + 1 Tbsp dried
cranberries): 5 grams of fibre

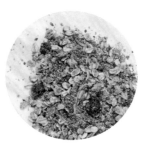

½ cup Maple Cinnamon
Granola (page 26):
7.8 grams of fibre

A Few Extra Tips & Tricks

AS A PROFESSIONAL HOME ECONOMIST, it's my job to try to make your life easier in the kitchen. Here are two of my favourite tips for jobs that can be messy or complicated.

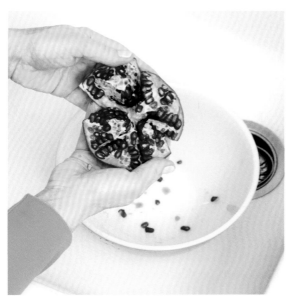
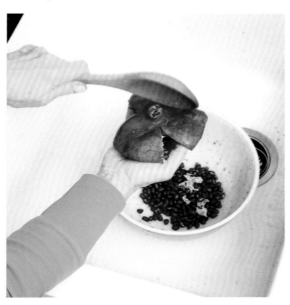

REMOVING POMEGRANATE SEEDS can be a pain, but with the method shown above and explained on page 104, you'll have a much easier time.

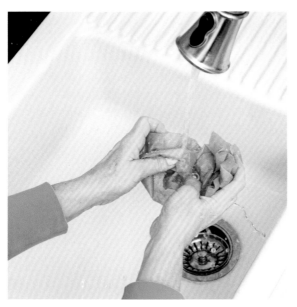
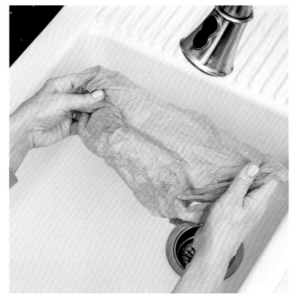

WETTING PARCHMENT PAPER, wringing it out and then using it will give you a more malleable piece that will meld into the pan without any trouble. It will also help minimize clean-up.

The Big Picture

MY MANTRA IS THAT A HEALTHY LIFESTYLE is a journey. You can start by adding more fibre to your diet, but that isn't the end of it. You need to add healthy habits to your day, every day. I'm not a fan of resolutions—you know, January 1 rolls around and you vow to lose 10 pounds, again. You're going to dust off your gym membership card, if you can even find it, and go for a walk every single day, rain or shine or in the dark of night, even when you'd rather be lounging on the couch watching reruns of *The Big Bang Theory* and eating day-old doughnuts.

The major glitch with resolutions is that they don't include the steps you need to take to reach your goals. So, keeping in mind that while my smaller goal is to get all of you eating a more fibre-rich diet, I'd also like you to start a healthy habit plan, the *Peace, Love & Fibre* way.

Here's how it works. Each month, pick one new habit from the list below. By the end of that month, your new healthy habit will be part of your new healthier lifestyle. As you work through my top 10 suggestions, find two more habits of your own. At the end of the year, you'll have developed at least 10, and possibly 12, new habits that will translate to a healthier, happier you.

1. BUMP UP YOUR VEGETABLES AND FRUIT

Mother Nature knew what she was doing when she created vegetables and fruit. These rock stars provide your body with disease-fighting antioxidants, soluble and insoluble fibre, vitamins, and minerals. People who eat seven to 10 servings of vegetables and fruit every day live longer, healthier lives. Start by adding one extra daily serving of vegetables or fruit for the first week. Every week after that, add one more daily serving. Every day, you should aim to eat one serving of leafy greens, one orange fruit or vegetable, and one apple.

GOAL: Four to six servings of vegetables per day and three to four servings of fruit per day.

2. WALK MORE

If there is a magic bullet for a long and healthy life, it's the big E-word: exercise. Our bodies are designed for movement, not for parking our butts in front of the computer or TV all day. Thirty minutes of walking (strolls don't count) make a huge impact on your long-term health. Though the common adage is "move it or lose it," I use "move it or you'll rust." It doesn't rhyme, but for me it's a great visual. Every week, add 10 more minutes of walking to your daily routine. Bonus: walking helps your brain and your butt.

GOAL: Thirty to 60 minutes of walking six or seven days a week.

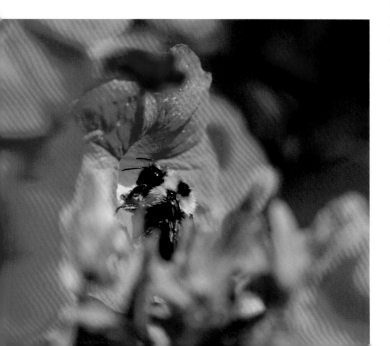

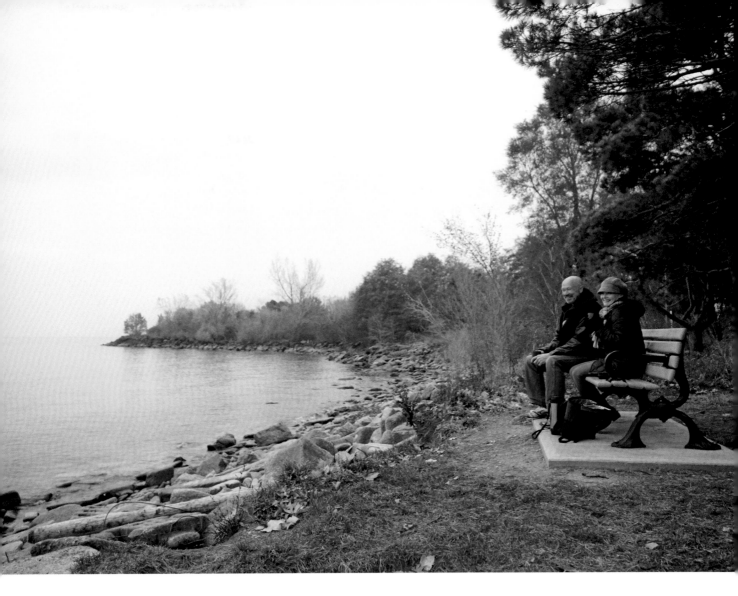

3. EAT FATTY FISH

Fatty fish don't have any fibre in them, but for long-term health, you need those valuable omega-3 fatty acids. Look for fish such as salmon, sardines, anchovies, herring, mackerel, or rainbow trout; all of them will help with brain function and help reduce your chances of having a heart attack or stroke. If you are eating one serving of fatty fish per week, add another. And serve fatty fish with any of my vegetable side dishes (pages 156 to 179) to increase your fibre intake.

GOAL: Two servings of fatty fish per week.

4. NURTURE RELATIONSHIPS

Strong social networks keep you young at heart. Most centenarians have rich social lives—take a page from their book and cultivate friendships from various age groups. You'll gain some new perspectives on life as well.

GOAL: Join a club or gym, meet friends for coffee, get involved with your church, or volunteer.

5. SWITCH TO WHOLE GRAINS

Ditch the white stuff and choose what your body really needs: whole grains. Switch from white or whole wheat bread to 100% whole grain whole wheat bread or 100% stone-milled whole wheat bread. Also switch from white rice to brown and from instant oats to whole grain oats or, better yet, steel-cut oats. When baking, add wheat germ to whole wheat flour or use stone-milled whole wheat flour. Try using spelt flour, whole grain barley, and whole grain oat flour as well.

GOAL: Toss out the refined grains and choose only whole grains.

6. KICK YOUR SWEET-TOOTH HABIT

Excess simple sugars can contribute to plaque buildup in your arteries, which can lead to heart disease. Simply switching from pop to water and eliminating that spoonful of sugar in your morning java can save your waistline from expanding and decrease your chances of having a heart attack or stroke. While you're at it, start eliminating sugary treats as well. As a bonus for menopausal women, this might help in the hot flash department too. If you need a treat, choose one from the Treats chapter (pages 180 to 221); the fibre content in these recipes will help your body deal with the extra sugar. But remember, they are still treats, to be eaten occasionally and enjoyed fully.

GOAL: Stop drinking sweetened drinks. If sweetened caffeinated drinks are your deal, eliminate one drink per day, as a rapid elimination of caffeinated drinks has been linked to caffeine withdrawal headaches.

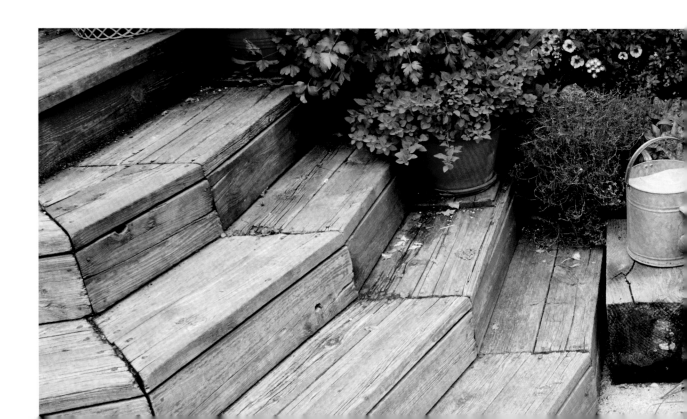

7. EAT NUTS

Eating a small handful of nuts every day will lower your chances of developing heart issues. All nuts contribute a different pedigree of power, so mix them up. Roughly, they all add about 3 to 6 grams of fibre per serving. Almonds, walnuts, pistachios, cashews, and peanuts are on my must-have list. Size really matters in this category—limit your nut intake to ¼ cup per day. Pack a serving as a portable snack.

GOAL: Have one serving of nuts four to seven times per week.

8. MAKE THE PULSE FAMILY YOUR FRIEND

Pulses, that wonderful family that includes beans, chickpeas, split peas, and lentils, are incredibly good for you. Adding them to your weekly eating routine is another healthy choice that pays big dividends down the road. Start by committing to one pulse meal a week. This cookbook is loaded with pulse recipes, so have fun exploring the options.

GOAL: By year's end, eat three to five pulse-based meals per week.

9. KEEP THE PRESSURE OFF

Managing stress is one of the most important ways to stay well. We all have stress in our lives, but the way in which each of us copes with it makes a difference. Learn to slow down your breathing if you start to feel stressed or anxious, and practise living in the moment and becoming more mindful of what you are doing.

GOAL: Become proactive about combatting stress by choosing an activity that calms you. I like yoga, meditation, tai chi, chi kung, walking, aerobic activities, and talking with friends.

10. PRACTISE KINDNESS

People who volunteer on a regular basis know that reaching out to others is a win-win. When we practise kindness, we are helping to heal this world. Hold the door for a senior, wave a driver in, smile, say thank you, visit your elderly relatives, or volunteer at a food bank. That act of kindness has a ripple effect and will bring happiness into your own life.

GOAL: Complete one kind act every day.

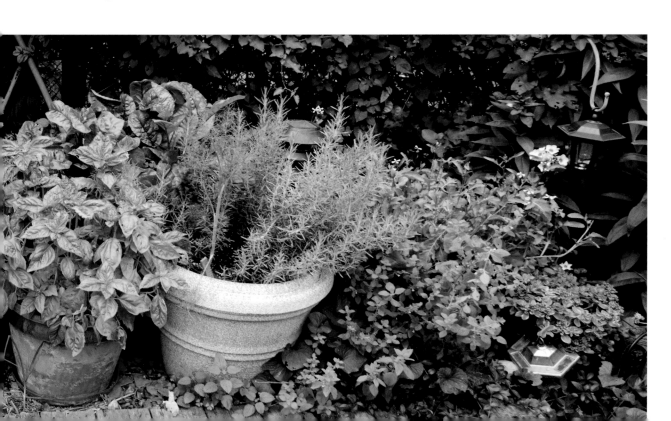

My Teacups & Me

MY DNA IS A FULL-ON CONCOCTION OF English and Scottish genes with a generous sprinkling of Irish chromosomes. Considering my genetic makeup is so entrenched in Britain and Ireland, I would be a scientific anomaly if I didn't love tea.

My gran and my great aunt Nell both made a brilliant cup of tea, and thankfully, they passed their skills down to me. With every cup of tea I sip, I'm paying tribute to them and to all the women in my life with whom I've shared a cup of tea.

My mom, although not a tea drinker herself, was the instigator of my obsession with teacups. She started collecting them when she was in her early 20s and she amassed quite the eclectic collection. At last count she had over 300 fine bone china beauties, which, sadly, she rarely used.

As a kid, I often wondered why anyone would collect such beautiful cups and saucers just to look at them. Yes, those teacups were very pretty, but they weren't ornaments—they were meant to be used. Whenever my mom wasn't home, I would sneak into the dining room and choose one of her treasures to make myself a wee pot of tea. I'd relish the secret moment, then wash, dry, and put the teacup back, making sure it was in the exact same place. I vowed that when I was a grown-up, I would use all my "good stuff" all the time.

True to my childhood vow, I do use all my good stuff. Too often, we save it for a special occasion, and then that special occasion never happens. Our good stuff lies around getting dusty. To my mind, keeping it in a cupboard doesn't honour it, nor does this honour ourselves. If you follow me on Instagram, you'll know that, to date, I have posted hundreds of pictures of my morning teacups with the hashtag #UseYourGoodStuff. And I want all of you to start using your good stuff too.

To me, teacups are so much more than vessels. They represent the peace and love in my life, the connection I feel with family and friends, and the drive I have to make this place a better world. I know it's a cliché, but life is short and you can't take your fancy china with you when you go! We need to find ways to celebrate every single day and discover joy in the little moments of our lives. Whether it's drinking from teacups, gardening, cooking, reading, meditating, or whatever floats your boat, I encourage you to take a few minutes each day to remind yourself that you're worth using the good stuff.

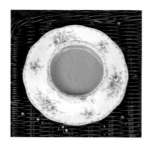

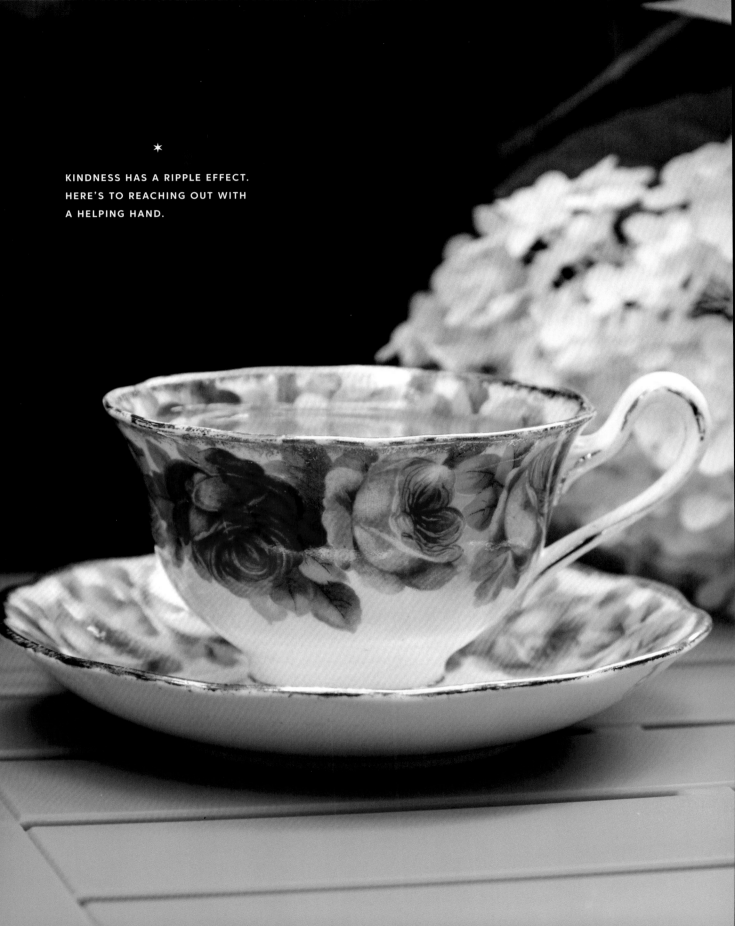

KINDNESS HAS A RIPPLE EFFECT.
HERE'S TO REACHING OUT WITH
A HELPING HAND.

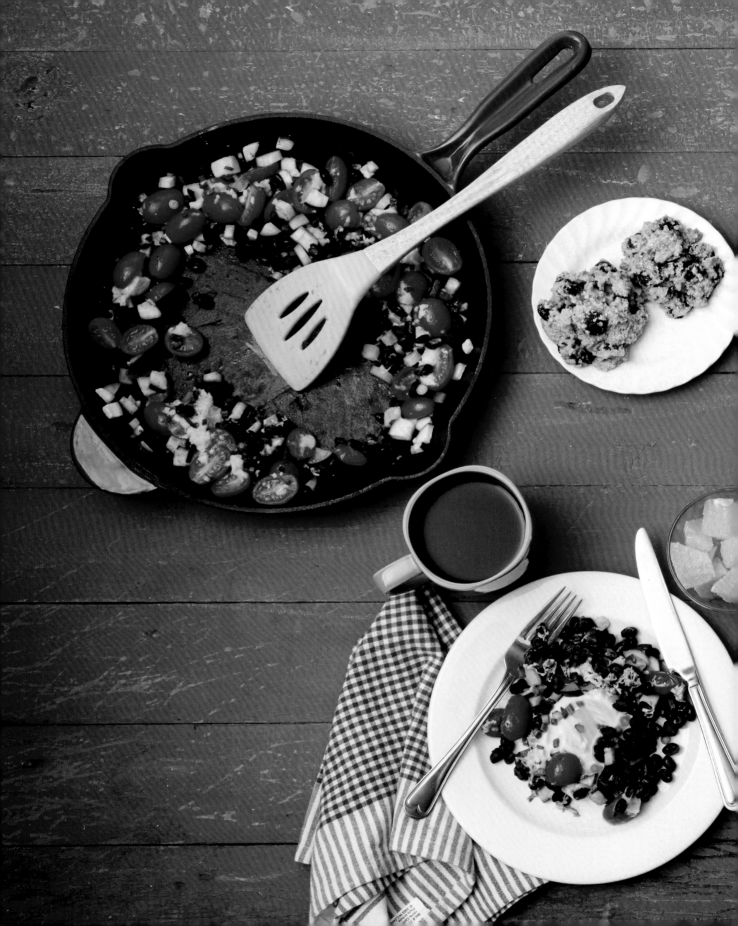

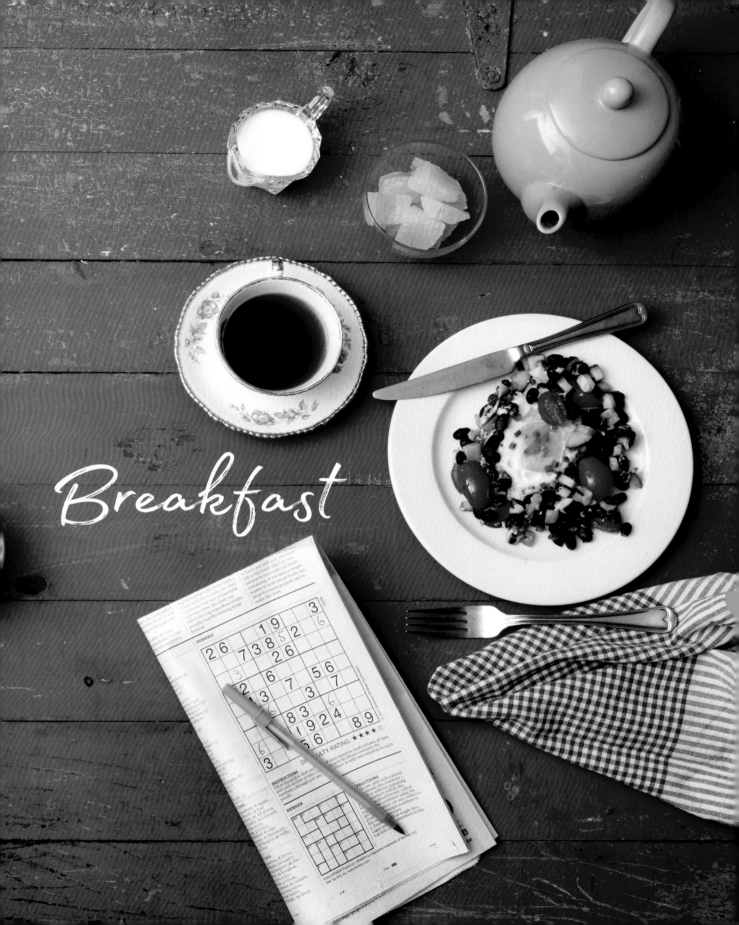

Breakfast

"To eat or not to eat breakfast" seems to be the debate of the decade. Do you eat breakfast or do you skip it? To add to the whole discussion, the *Wall Street Journal* reported in April 2017 that there was a trend toward eating not one, but two breakfasts every day. With an epidemic of obesity knocking on our doors, who came up with that ridiculous plan?

Has breakfast become a marketing campaign to encourage us to buy certain foods and eat them first thing in the morning, or is eating breakfast a must for our long-term health? Let's look at some facts. In a study published in January 2017 in *Circulation*, the American Heart Association's journal, researchers at Columbia University gave two big cheers for breakfast eating. Their findings included the following:

- Breakfast eaters were less likely than breakfast abstainers to have high blood pressure and high cholesterol.

- Breakfast eaters didn't tend to snack or graze throughout the day as much as the breakfast abstainers did, and the latter were more likely to become obese and/ or be diagnosed with type 2 diabetes.

The researchers also stated that how often a person ate was linked to the risk factors that can lead to heart disease, high blood pressure, high blood sugar levels, and a reduction in the body's ability to regulate insulin. Translation: nibbling all day isn't a great plan of attack. Skipping breakfast can lead to all-day nibbles, and that can also lead to weight gain.

I know we're all busy. We're multitasking every morning: packing lunches, getting kids off to school, getting ready for work, walking the dog—the list of reasons for not eating breakfast is endless. But as a professional home economist, it's my job to offer solutions.

Here's how I tackle the breakfast dilemma. First and foremost, I look at breakfast as a way to recharge my brain, get my body going, get in those much-needed grams of fibre, and help set the tone for my day. It starts with my positive attitude about the first meal of the day. My wonderfully optimistic dad, who lived to be 94 years old, always planned what he was going to have for breakfast before he even got out of bed. I loved his style.

Like my dad, I plan my breakfast, but I base my choices on my mood, how pressed I am for time, and the season. If it's a gorgeous, sunny day and I'm not in a hurry, my breakfast is a bowl of Greek yogurt with seasonal berries, fruit, or Honey-Roasted Apricots (page 55), as well as walnuts, ground flaxseed, and maybe a small handful of my Maple Cinnamon Granola (page 26). See the picture of me enjoying that breakfast on my front porch on page 27? I'm smiling because eating breakfast puts me in a good mood, which is great news for my husband and son. Late for work? I grab three of Mairlyn's Energy Balls (page 52) and a travel cup of tea, and I'm gone. Winter weekend brunch? I might start the day off with Mayan Hot Cocoa (page 37), and then an hour later make Morning Eggs Mexican-Style (page 50).

Whatever you choose, make it a habit to eat something healthy before you begin your day or

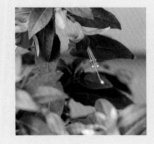

fly out the door. Breakfast can send you out into the world with a positive attitude affecting not only you but also the people you encounter throughout your day. It's a win-win.

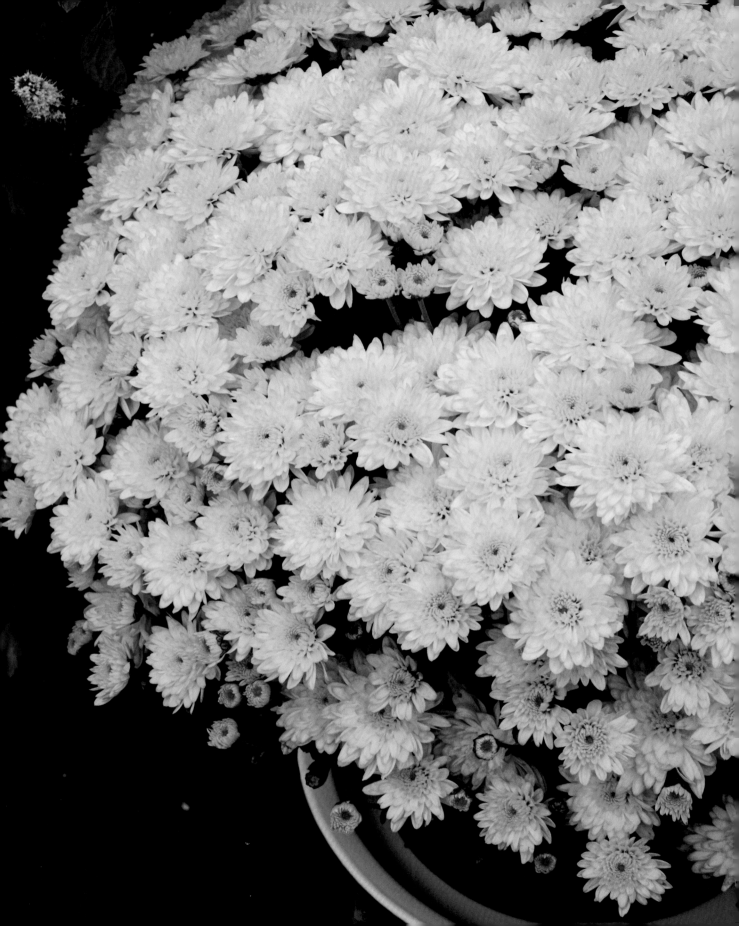

Maple Cinnamon Granola VEG LF · *Makes 7 cups*

MOST STORE-BOUGHT GRANOLAS ARE LADEN WITH SUGAR AND FAT. Nutritionally speaking, they're more like crumbled cookies disguised as a health food. Check out the nutrient breakdown on this granola—and don't let the fat grams scare you off. Research tells us that it's not the number of grams of fat that we should be concerned about, but rather the quality of those grams. The fat in flaxseed, which is where most of the fat is coming from here, is heart-healthy. The other source of fat is from canola oil, also heart-healthy. Now that doesn't give you carte blanche to go crazy and eat a huge portion; a ½ cup is all you get. But enjoy each bite. Your heart is thanking you.

4 cups large oat flakes

1 cup oat bran

1 cup natural wheat germ

2 tsp ground cinnamon

¼ cup pure amber maple syrup

3 Tbsp canola oil

2 tsp pure vanilla extract

1 cup ground flaxseed
(see page 184)

½ cup dried cranberries

1 SERVING = ½ CUP
PER SERVING: 274 CALORIES, 10.2 G TOTAL
FAT, 1.2 G SATURATED FAT, 0 G TRANS FAT,
0 MG CHOLESTEROL, 5 MG SODIUM,
40.9 G CARBOHYDRATE, 7.8 G FIBRE,
6.8 G SUGARS, 5.9 G ADDED SUGARS,
9.2 G PROTEIN, 310 MG POTASSIUM
CARBOHYDRATE CHOICE = 2 CHOICES

1. Adjust the racks in the oven so that one rack is in the middle of the oven and the other rack is just above. Preheat the oven to 275°F. Line two large rimmed baking sheets with parchment paper. Set aside.

2. In a large bowl, toss together the oat flakes, oat bran, wheat germ, and cinnamon. Using a glass measuring cup so that it's easier to pour, measure out the maple syrup, then add the oil and vanilla to the cup, whisk quickly, and drizzle evenly over the oat mixture. Using clean hands, massage or rub the maple syrup mixture into the oats to coat all the ingredients. Divide equally between your baking sheets and spread out evenly. Don't wash the bowl yet.

3. Place one sheet on the top rack of the oven and the other on the middle rack and bake for 10 minutes. Remove the baking sheets from the oven and stir, making sure that you spread out the mixture evenly in the pans once again. Place the sheet that was on the middle rack on the top rack, and vice versa. Bake for 10 minutes.

4. Remove from the oven and stir. Return the baking sheets to the oven, once again switching their positions. Bake for 10 more minutes. Remove from the oven and stir, then return to the oven, changing positions again, and bake for 10 more minutes. (Yes, there is a lot of repositioning going on, but you don't want the granola to burn—I've got your back.) For anyone counting, that's a total of 40 minutes of cooking time.

5. Remove the baking sheets from the oven and divide the flaxseed equally over each sheet. Stir well. Pop back into the oven, reversing the position of the sheets for the last time. Bake 5 to 10 minutes more, until the oats are golden brown and your house smells like warm oat cookies. Remove from the oven and transfer the granola back into the large bowl that hopefully you didn't wash. Add the cranberries and toss well.

6. Return to the baking sheets, dividing equally and spreading the granola out so it will cool completely. Once completely cool, store in a large glass jar or a container with a tight-fitting lid for up to 1 month.

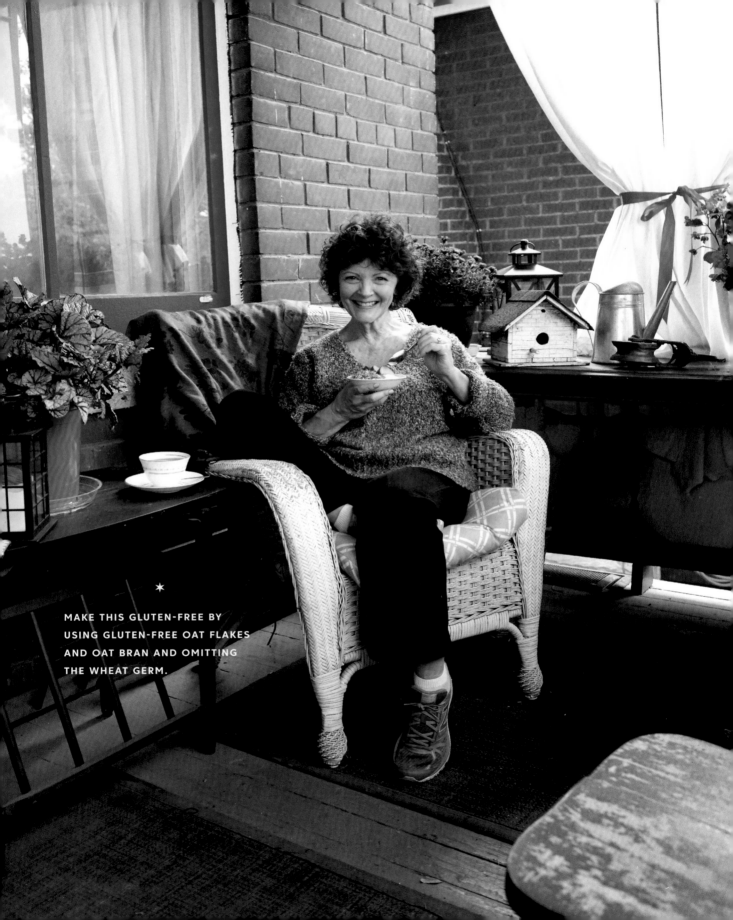

MAKE THIS GLUTEN-FREE BY
USING GLUTEN-FREE OAT FLAKES
AND OAT BRAN AND OMITTING
THE WHEAT GERM.

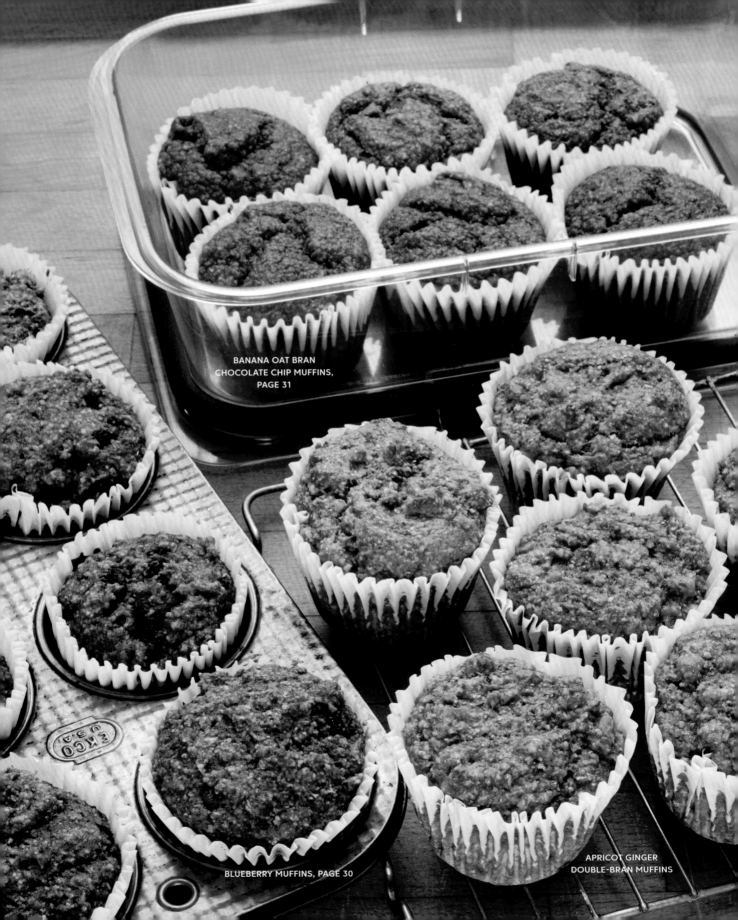

BANANA OAT BRAN
CHOCOLATE CHIP MUFFINS,
PAGE 31

BLUEBERRY MUFFINS, PAGE 30

APRICOT GINGER
DOUBLE-BRAN MUFFINS

Apricot Ginger Double-Bran Muffins VEG · *Makes 12 muffins*

THESE DOUBLE-BRAN MUFFINS GET THEIR FIBRE CLOUT FROM OAT AND WHEAT BRAN PLUS the super-fibre star—ladies and gentlemen, put your hands together for lentils. Before you ask "what are lentils doing in a muffin?" keep in mind that they're puréed, so only the cook will know about them. Okay, your colon will ring in, but when you serve them, mum's the word.

WET INGREDIENTS

1 cup canned lentils, rinsed and well drained (see note)

2 cups 1% buttermilk

½ cup whole walnuts

1 cup packed whole dried apricots

½ cup oat bran

½ cup coarsely chopped dried candied ginger (see note on page 200)

½ cup packed dark brown sugar

1 omega-3 egg

1 Tbsp pure vanilla extract

DRY INGREDIENTS

1 cup whole wheat flour

¾ cup ground flaxseed (see page 184)

½ cup wheat bran

2 Tbsp natural wheat germ

1 tsp ground cinnamon

1 tsp baking powder

1 tsp baking soda

NOTE: One 19 fl oz (540 mL) can of lentils is just shy of 2 cups. Toss the leftover lentils into a green salad.

1. Place a rack in the middle of the oven and preheat the oven to 375°F. Line a 12-cup muffin pan with extra-large or jumbo paper liners; these babies are big. Set aside.

2. Prepare the wet ingredients. In a large food processor fitted with the blade attachment, pulse the lentils and buttermilk until you can't recognize the lentils. Then add the walnuts, apricots, oat bran, ginger, sugar, egg, and vanilla. Pulse until the apricots are the size of chickpeas. Don't go crazy pushing the pulse button and turning this mixture into a smoothie. It should have small visible pieces of walnuts, apricots, and dried candied ginger. Let sit for at least 10 minutes. This helps the oat bran absorb some of the liquid.

3. Pulse the wet ingredients once more and then add the dry ingredients: the flour, flaxseed, wheat bran, wheat germ, cinnamon, baking powder, and baking soda. Pulse gently until there are no visible dry ingredients. This should take four to six pulses.

4. Using a ¼-cup ice-cream scoop with a release button, scoop out a heaping ¼ cup of the batter and fill each of the muffin cups. You are going to be tempted to make more than 12 muffins, but stop yourself. These muffins don't rise as much as those made with refined flour. What you see is pretty much what you'll get after they're baked.

5. Bake for 22 to 24 minutes or until a toothpick inserted in the centre of a muffin comes out clean.

6. Let the muffins cool in the pan on a wire rack for 2 minutes. Remove the muffins from the pan and let them cool completely on the rack. Store the muffins in an airtight container for up to 2 days or in the freezer for up to 2 months.

1 SERVING = 1 MUFFIN
PER SERVING: 254 CALORIES, 7.7 G TOTAL FAT, 1.1 G SATURATED FAT, 0 G TRANS FAT, 18 MG CHOLESTEROL, 253 MG SODIUM, 39.4 G CARBOHYDRATE, 5.9 G FIBRE, 23 G SUGARS, 16.1 G ADDED SUGARS, 8.2 G PROTEIN, 519 MG POTASSIUM
CARBOHYDRATE CHOICE = 2 CHOICES

Blueberry Muffins VEG · *Makes 12 muffins*

GROWING UP, I ATE ONLY CONVENTIONALLY GROWN BLUEBERRIES—I didn't know what a wild blueberry was until I moved to Toronto. Harvested by hand in the wilds of Ontario, Quebec, and the Maritimes, these sweet little gems are fabulous, albeit expensive—though worth every blessed penny. I prefer wild blueberries as they are. Baking them just seems like a blueberry tragedy. Having said that, use whichever fresh seasonal blueberry you love in this recipe.

WET INGREDIENTS

1 cup canned lentils, rinsed and well drained (see note on page 29)

1 cup 1% buttermilk

¾ cup packed dark brown sugar

½ cup oat bran

1 omega-3 egg

DRY INGREDIENTS

1 cup whole wheat flour

¾ cup flaxseed meal (see page 184)

2 Tbsp natural wheat germ

1 Tbsp ground cinnamon

1 Tbsp lemon or orange zest

2 tsp baking powder

1 tsp baking soda

2 cups fresh (not frozen) local blueberries, rinsed and patted dry

1. Place a rack in the middle of the oven and preheat the oven to 375°F. Line a 12-cup muffin pan with extra-large or jumbo paper liners. Set aside.

2. Prepare the wet ingredients. In a large bowl with a hand-held immersion blender or in a stand blender, purée the lentils and buttermilk until you can't recognize the lentils. Pour into a medium bowl and whisk in the brown sugar, oat bran, and egg. (You're probably thinking brown sugar and oat bran aren't wet ingredients. And you'd be right. In this recipe, they need to be added to the *true* wet ingredients so they can absorb some of the liquid before adding them to the dry ingredients.)

3. In another medium bowl, whisk together the dry ingredients: flour, flaxseed meal, wheat germ, cinnamon, zest, baking powder, and baking soda.

4. Pour the dry ingredients into the wet ingredients. Stir together using a rubber spatula or a large wooden spoon. Gently fold in the blueberries.

5. Using a ¼-cup ice-cream scoop with a release button, scoop out a heaping ¼ cup of the batter and fill each of the muffin cups. You are going to be tempted to make more than 12 muffins, but don't even think about it. The muffins won't rise very much due to the whole grains and dense fibre-rich ingredients we're using.

6. Bake for 23 to 25 minutes or until a toothpick inserted in the centre of a muffin comes out clean. Cool in the pan on a wire rack for 2 minutes. Remove the muffins from the pan and let them cool completely on the rack. Store in an airtight container for up to 2 days or in the freezer for up to 3 months.

1 SERVING = 1 MUFFIN
PER SERVING: 193 CALORIES, 4.6 G TOTAL FAT, 0.7 G SATURATED FAT, 0 G TRANS FAT, 17 MG CHOLESTEROL, 237 MG SODIUM, 30.3 G CARBOHYDRATE, 4.7 G FIBRE, 16.8 G SUGARS, 14.1 G ADDED SUGARS, 6.2 G PROTEIN, 257 MG POTASSIUM
CARBOHYDRATE CHOICE = 2 CHOICES

Banana Oat Bran Chocolate Chip Muffins VEG · *Makes 12 muffins*

HISTORICALLY, THE SCOTS WERE KNOWN AS FIERCE WARRIORS, often running naked into battle. One theory as to why they were such ferocious fighters is that they lived on barren land and needed their natural resources for survival, fighting to the death for them. Extremely valid, but my theory is that it was all the oats they ate. Hear me out: oats act as an anti-inflammatory and are heart-healthy, plus the soluble fibre helps remove toxins from the body—all important attributes for surviving in a harsh land and running naked into battle.

WET INGREDIENTS

1 cup 1% buttermilk

1½ cups oat bran

1½ cups thawed and mashed frozen ripe bananas (3 to 4)

¼ cup canola oil

½ cup packed dark brown sugar

1 omega-3 egg

2 tsp pure vanilla extract

DRY INGREDIENTS

1¼ cups whole wheat flour

2 Tbsp natural cocoa powder

2 Tbsp natural wheat germ

2 tsp ground cinnamon

1 tsp baking powder

1 tsp baking soda

¼ cup dark chocolate chips

1. Place a rack in the middle of the oven and preheat the oven to 375°F. Line a 12-cup muffin pan with extra-large or jumbo paper liners. Set aside.

2. In a large bowl, whisk together the wet ingredients: buttermilk, oat bran, bananas, oil, brown sugar, egg, and vanilla. Set aside.

3. In a medium bowl, whisk together the dry ingredients: flour, cocoa powder, wheat germ, cinnamon, baking powder, and baking soda. Stir in the chocolate chips.

4. Add the dry ingredients to the wet ingredients and mix to combine, using either a large wooden spoon or a large spatula. You can't theoretically overmix these, but don't go crazy with it.

5. Using a ¼-cup ice-cream scoop with a release button, scoop out a heaping ¼ cup of the batter and fill each of the muffin cups. You'll want to make more than 12, but all my whole grain muffins make 12 large muffins.

6. Bake for 23 to 25 minutes or until a toothpick inserted in the centre of a muffin comes out clean.

7. Let the muffins cool in the pan on a wire rack for 2 minutes. Remove the muffins from the pan and let them cool completely on the rack. Store in an airtight container for up to 2 days or in the freezer for up to 2 months.

1 SERVING = 1 MUFFIN
PER SERVING: 231 CALORIES, 8.6 G TOTAL FAT, 1.8 G SATURATED FAT, 0 G TRANS FAT, 17 MG CHOLESTEROL, 189 MG SODIUM, 30.4 G CARBOHYDRATE, 4.1 G FIBRE, 15.3 G SUGARS, 10.3 G ADDED SUGARS, 6.4 G PROTEIN, 318 MG POTASSIUM
CARBOHYDRATE CHOICE = 2 CHOICES

Overnight Steel-Cut Oats Three Ways

A COUPLE OF YEARS AGO, overnight oats were one of the biggest food trends on social media. You couldn't go onto any platform without seeing hundreds of food-porn pictures of overnight oats in 2-cup canning or mason jars.

I didn't buy into the hype, but after being bombarded by endless pictures, I finally gave in. I put on my food scientist hat and tried several recipes. Sadly, none were as tasty as the pictures made them appear to be, nor did the recipes do justice to steel-cut oats. I'm sure some recipes out there were fabulous, but I didn't find any in my research. It could be my dislike of raw steel-cut oats, or maybe I'm not a big fan of raw oat flakes, or maybe I was being super picky. Whatever the reason, it spurred me to create my own spins on overnight oats.

Tips Before You Start

- Unless you love super-chewy steel-cut oats, assemble these 10 to 12 hours before you want to eat them. Counting backward from when you normally eat breakfast, do the math and you'll know when to start them.
- The recipes range from 10.4 grams of fibre to a whopping 16 grams of fibre per serving. Choose according to your fibre needs.

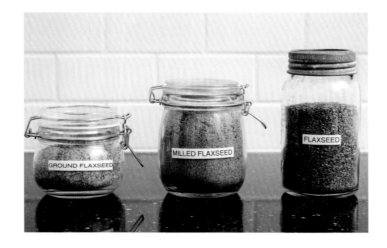

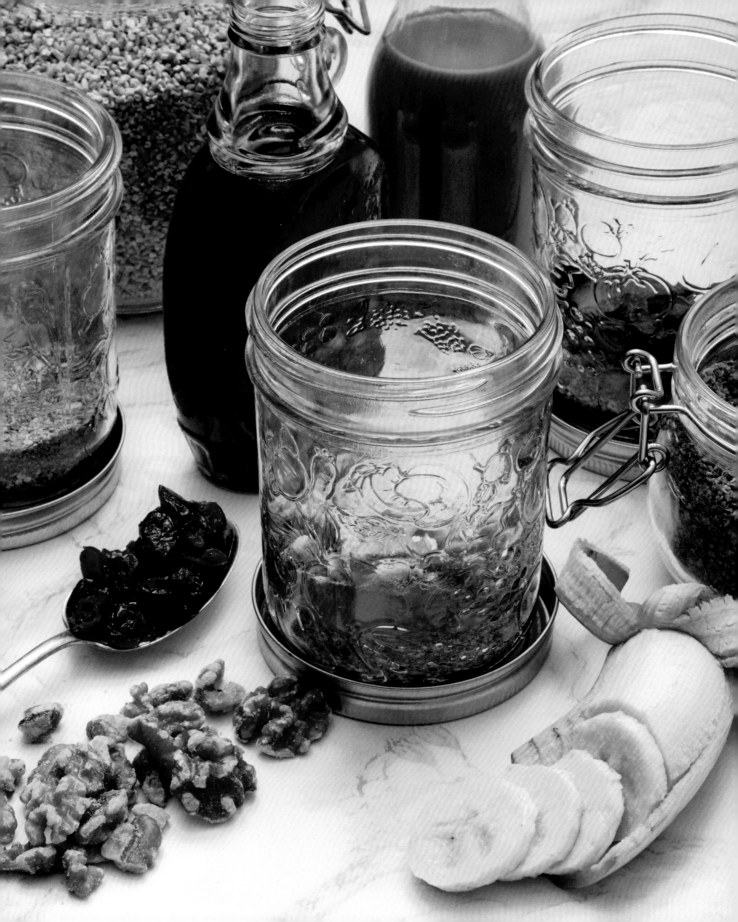

TRADITIONAL OVERNIGHT OATS FOR THE STEEL-CUT PURISTS VEG · *Serves 1*

¼ cup steel-cut oats

2 Tbsp ground flaxseed
(see page 184)

2 Tbsp dried cranberries

¾ cup skim milk or soy beverage

1 Tbsp pure amber maple syrup

1 tsp pure vanilla extract

½ tsp ground cinnamon

2 Tbsp whole walnuts

1. Spoon all the ingredients, except the walnuts, into a 2-cup mason jar with a screw-top lid. Screw on the lid and shake vigorously. You can either add the walnuts at this stage or wait to add them the next day, after the oats have been cooked. The walnuts won't be as firm if you add them at the beginning of the recipe. Store the jar overnight in the fridge.

2. In the morning, give the jar another vigorous shake, remove the lid, and place in the microwave. Heat on high and stir in the following order: 1 minute, stir, 1 minute, stir, 40 seconds, stir. Remove from the microwave, stir, and cover for 15 minutes while you run around getting ready for your day. When you're ready to eat, stir in the walnuts if you haven't added them already, and enjoy.

1 SERVING = 1 RECIPE
PER SERVING: 507 CALORIES, 18.3 G TOTAL FAT, 1.8 G SATURATED FAT, 0 G TRANS FAT,
3 MG CHOLESTEROL, 88 MG SODIUM, 72.7 G CARBOHYDRATE, 10.4 G FIBRE, 33.9 G SUGARS,
20.3 G ADDED SUGARS, 18 G PROTEIN, 703 MG POTASSIUM
CARBOHYDRATE CHOICE = 4 CHOICES

CHOCOLATE BANANA WALNUT OVERNIGHT OATS VEG · *Serves 1*

¼ cup steel-cut oats

2 Tbsp ground flaxseed
(see page 184)

2 Tbsp natural cocoa powder

¾ cup skim milk or soy beverage

1 to 2 Tbsp pure amber maple
syrup

1 tsp pure vanilla extract

½ ripe banana, thinly sliced

2 Tbsp whole walnuts

1 SERVING = 1 RECIPE
PER SERVING: 533 CALORIES, 19.7 G TOTAL
FAT, 2.6 G SATURATED FAT, 0 G TRANS FAT,
3 MG CHOLESTEROL, 91 MG SODIUM,
78.5 G CARBOHYDRATE, 13.9 G FIBRE,
31.3 G SUGARS, 12.5 G ADDED SUGARS,
21.5 G PROTEIN, 1066 MG POTASSIUM
CARBOHYDRATE CHOICE = 4 CHOICES

1. Spoon all the ingredients, except the banana and walnuts, into a 2-cup mason jar with a screw-top lid. Screw on the lid and shake vigorously. If the cocoa powder hasn't dissolved, shake it again. You can either add the banana and walnuts here or wait to add them the next day, after the oats have been cooked. They won't be as firm if you add them at the beginning of the recipe. Store the jar overnight in the fridge.

2. In the morning, give the jar another vigorous shake, remove the lid, and place in the microwave. Heat on high and stir in the following order: 1 minute, stir, 1 minute, stir, 40 seconds, stir. Remove the jar from the microwave, stir, and add the sliced banana, if you didn't add it the night before (see note). Cover for 15 minutes while you perform your morning routines. When you're ready to eat, stir in the walnuts if you haven't already, and enjoy.

NOTE: The banana really softens when you add it before the oats sit. If you want the texture of the banana to be firmer, add it when you add the walnuts (if you haven't added them the night before).

CHOCOLATE ALMOND OVERNIGHT OATS FOR ALMOND LOVERS VEG · *Serves 1*

¼ cup steel-cut oats

2 Tbsp ground flaxseed
(see page 184)

1 Tbsp natural cocoa powder

1 cup chocolate almond
beverage

1 Tbsp dark or bittersweet
chocolate chips

1 Tbsp pure amber maple syrup
(optional)

1 tsp pure vanilla extract

2 Tbsp whole almonds

✳

OLD-SCHOOL STEEL-CUT OATS

Still love making a pot of
steel-cut oats from scratch on
a cold winter morning? Make
that regular pot of steel-cut
oats according to the directions,
then add per serving: 2 Tbsp
dried cranberries, 1 Tbsp
ground flaxseed, ¼ cup whole
walnuts, and a sprinkle of
ground cinnamon. Your regular
bowl of steel-cut oats just
went from 4 grams of fibre
to 8.2 grams.

1. Spoon all the ingredients, except the almonds, into a 2-cup mason
   jar with a screw-top lid. Screw on the lid and shake vigorously;
   you want to make sure the cocoa powder dissolves. You can either
   add the almonds here or wait to add them the next day, after the
   oats are cooked. They won't be as firm if you add them at the
   beginning of the recipe. Store the jar overnight in the fridge.

2. In the morning, give the jar a vigorous shake, remove the lid, and
   place in the microwave. Heat on high and stir in the following
   order: 1 minute, stir, 1 minute, stir, 40 seconds, stir. Remove the
   jar from the microwave, stir, and cover for 15 minutes while you
   multitask through your morning routine. When you're ready
   to eat, stir in the almonds if you haven't added them already,
   and enjoy.

1 SERVING = 1 RECIPE
PER SERVING: 533 CALORIES, 25.7 G TOTAL FAT, 5 G SATURATED FAT, 0 G TRANS FAT,
0 MG CHOLESTEROL, 158 MG SODIUM, 67.6 G CARBOHYDRATE, 16 G FIBRE, 22.4 G SUGARS,
21.2 G ADDED SUGARS, 15.1 G PROTEIN, 805 MG POTASSIUM
CARBOHYDRATE CHOICE = 3½ CHOICES

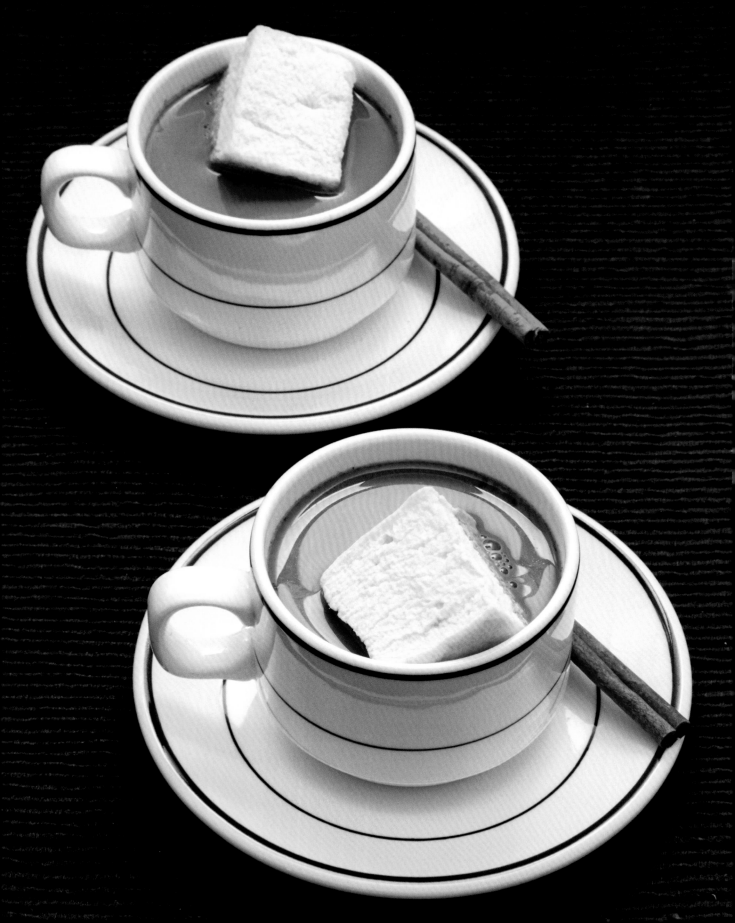

Mayan Hot Cocoa for Two   VEG · *Serves 2*

I HAVE SEVERAL FOOD ISSUES THAT REALLY GET ME RANTING, and one is when I hear people use "hot chocolate" and "cocoa" interchangeably. Cocoa and hot chocolate are two very different beverages. Cocoa is made with fibre-rich, heart-healthy cocoa powder and hot chocolate is made with melted chocolate, which has less fibre and way more fat. Both are super-yum and a great way to get a chocolate fix and add some calcium and magnesium into your diet. This spicy cocoa is based on a spicy hot chocolate recipe I tried at Soma, a high-end chocolate factory and retail store in Toronto. It feels like a big warm hug in a mug.

2 cups 1% milk

¼ cup natural cocoa powder

¼ cup liquid honey, granulated sugar, or sweetener of your choice

¼ tsp ground ginger

¼ tsp ground cinnamon

⅛ tsp red pepper flakes

1 Tbsp pure vanilla extract

NOTE: If you really need a treat, I give you full permission to add a marshmallow and use a cinnamon stick as a stir stick, just like in the picture. Just keep in mind that marshmallows are not vegetarian.

1. Heat the milk in a small pot over medium heat, or in the microwave on high, until steamy. On the stove, this should take 5 to 6 minutes; in the microwave, it will take 2 to 3 minutes.

2. Whisk in the cocoa powder, honey or other sweetener, ginger, cinnamon, red pepper flakes, and vanilla until the cocoa has dissolved and the mixture is hot. Divide between two mugs and serve.

1 SERVING = ½ RECIPE WITHOUT A MARSHMALLOW, MADE WITH HONEY
PER SERVING: 255 CALORIES, 3.9 G TOTAL FAT, 2.4 G SATURATED FAT, 0 G TRANS FAT, 14 MG CHOLESTEROL, 117 MG SODIUM, 46.9 G CARBOHYDRATE, 4.2 G FIBRE, 40.9 G SUGARS, 27.2 G ADDED SUGARS, 10.8 G PROTEIN, 566 MG POTASSIUM
CARBOHYDRATE CHOICE = 3 CHOICES

Lemon Ricotta Pancakes VEG · *Serves 4*

MOST WEEKENDS IN THE SUMMER, MY HUSBAND AND I HEAD UP NORTH to stay at my BFF Michale and her husband's cottage in Muskoka, Ontario. I bring up tons of food, she has tons of food—it's basically a food extravaganza. We both follow the inspiring and beautiful posts from Calgary home economist Sylvia Kong on Instagram @savory.palate. One weekend, we had a hankering for lemon ricotta pancakes, having both seen Sylvia's pancake post, which was inspired by a *Looneyspoons* recipe. Here's my fibre spin on it, with Michale's idea of adding raspberries instead of blueberries because we didn't have any blueberries at the cottage and no one wanted to drive into town to get them. Check out the nutrient breakdown before you scarf down eight of these delicious pancakes. One serving of four pancakes has 21.5 grams of protein and a whopping 14.9 grams of fibre, so it's a meal all by itself.

1 cup fresh (not frozen) local raspberries or blueberries

DRY INGREDIENTS

1¾ cups whole grain barley flour

½ cup flaxseed meal
(see page 184)

3 Tbsp granulated sugar

1 Tbsp baking powder

1 tsp baking soda

Zest of 1 lemon

WET INGREDIENTS

3 Tbsp fresh lemon juice

1 cup smooth low-fat ricotta

1¼ cups skim milk

2 omega-3 eggs

2 Tbsp canola oil

1 tsp pure vanilla extract

1 Tbsp oil for the skillet (divided)

Icing sugar, for serving, optional

**1 SERVING = 4 PANCAKES WITHOUT
ICING SUGAR**
PER SERVING: 547 CALORIES, 21 G TOTAL FAT,
5.1 G SATURATED FAT, 0 G TRANS FAT,
118 MG CHOLESTEROL, 739 MG SODIUM,
67.3 G CARBOHYDRATE, 14.9 G FIBRE,
16.1 G SUGARS, 9.6 G ADDED SUGARS,
21.5 G PROTEIN, 627 MG POTASSIUM
CARBOHYDRATE CHOICE = 3½ CHOICES

1. Gently rinse the berries and lay them on a clean tea towel or paper towel to air-dry.

2. Place a rack in the middle of the oven and preheat the oven to 200°F. Line a large rimmed baking sheet with parchment paper and set aside.

3. Prepare the dry ingredients. In a large bowl, whisk together the flour, flaxseed meal, sugar, baking powder, baking soda, and lemon zest.

4. Prepare the wet ingredients. In a medium bowl, whisk together the lemon juice, ricotta, milk, eggs, oil, and vanilla.

5. Heat a 12- or 14-inch non-stick skillet or a griddle over medium heat. Use a pastry brush to lightly coat with a tiny bit of oil, saving the rest for the remaining batches.

6. Add the wet ingredients to the dry ingredients and use a large wooden spoon to gently mix.

7. Pour ¼ cup of the batter into the hot pan to form a 4-inch pancake. You will probably fit three pancakes per pan, unless it's a huge griddle, in which case, I'm slightly jealous. Pop three or four berries on top of each pancake.

8. The pancakes will be ready to flip when the undersides are golden brown and the tops look slightly cooked with the odd open bubble, 3 to 4 minutes. Flip and cook the pancakes for an additional 3 to 5 minutes, until the undersides are golden and the centres spring back when pressed. Place cooked pancakes on the prepared baking sheet in the oven to keep warm while you cook the remaining batches.

9. Serve each pancake with a sprinkling of ¼ tsp icing sugar if desired.

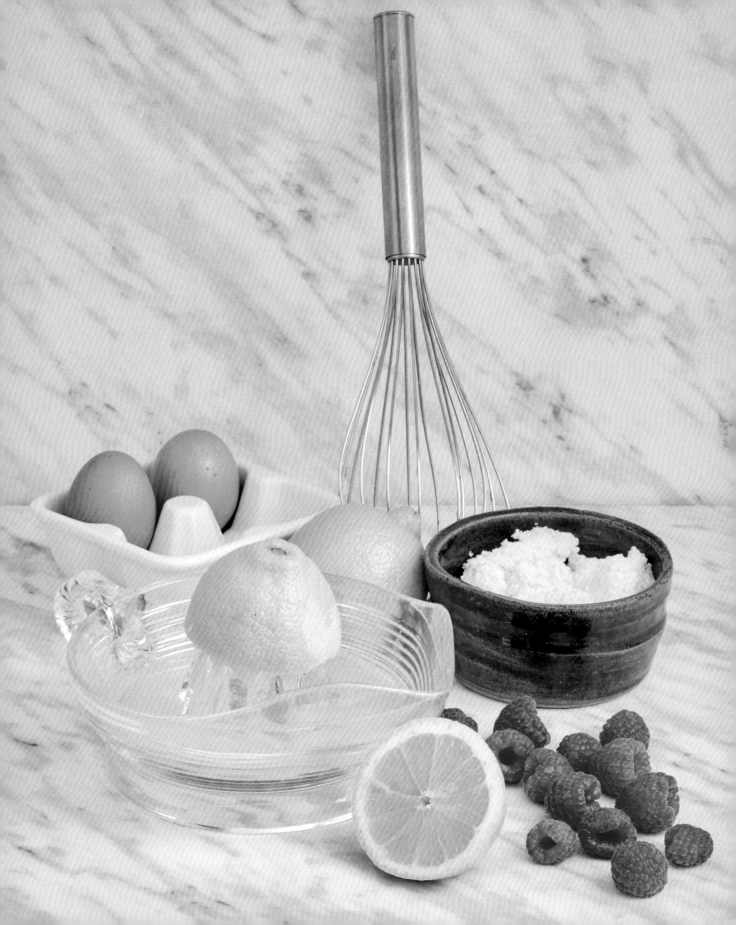

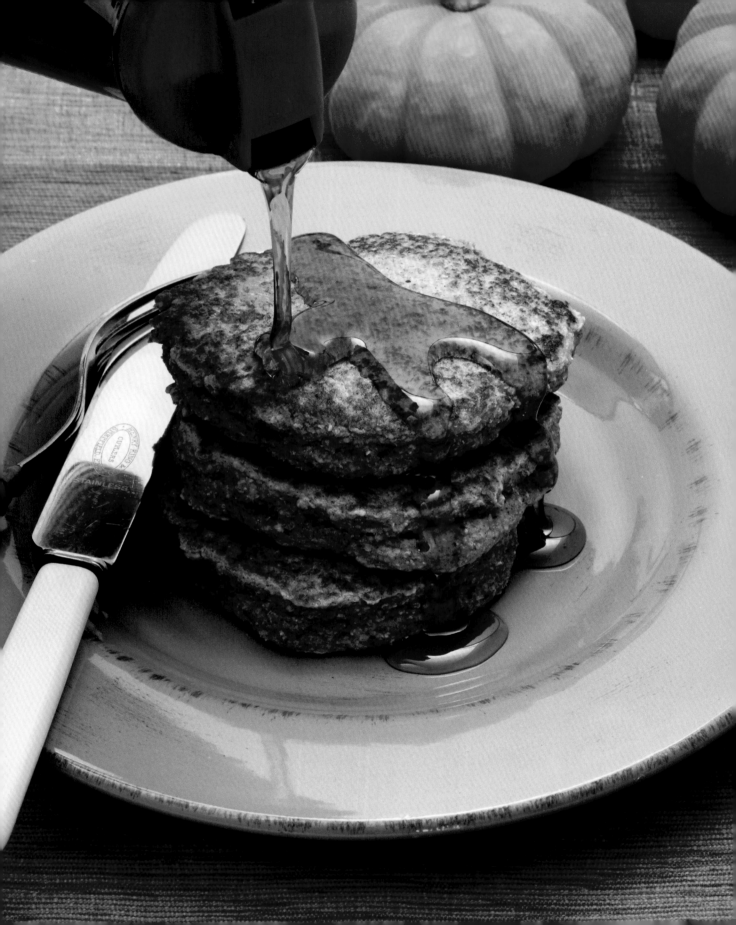

Pumpkin Spice Griddle Cakes VEG LF · *Serves 6*

TO ME, FALL AND PUMPKINS ARE INEXTRICABLY LINKED. I'm a visual person, so when the leaves start turning, I get a hankering for all things orange and I start eating squash and pumpkin. These pumpkin griddle cakes, thicker and more cake-like than their pancake cousins, hit the spot on a Saturday morning in October along with a big pot of chai.

WET INGREDIENTS

1¾ cups almond beverage

1½ cups pure pumpkin purée (see note)

1 cup oat bran

2 omega-3 eggs

2 Tbsp pure amber maple syrup or liquid honey, plus extra for serving

DRY INGREDIENTS

1¼ cups whole wheat flour

¼ cup natural wheat germ

1 Tbsp baking powder

2 tsp ground cinnamon

¼ tsp ground nutmeg

¼ tsp ground ginger

¼ tsp ground allspice

⅛ tsp ground cloves

1 Tbsp canola oil for the skillet (divided)

NOTE: Pure pumpkin purée and pumpkin pie filling are totally different entities. The recipes in this cookbook call for pure pumpkin purée, which is made from squash and pumpkin or just pumpkin, and nothing else. Pumpkin pie filling has added sugars and spices and will ruin any recipe that calls for the pure stuff.

1. In a large bowl, whisk together the wet ingredients: almond beverage, pumpkin purée, oat bran, eggs, and maple syrup or honey. Set aside for at least 5 minutes and up to 10 minutes so the oat bran can absorb some of the liquid.

2. Meanwhile, in a small bowl, whisk together the dry ingredients: flour, wheat germ, baking powder, cinnamon, nutmeg, ginger, allspice, and cloves.

3. Preheat the oven to 200°F. Line a large rimmed baking sheet with parchment paper and set aside.

4. Add the dry ingredients to the wet ingredients and stir well until all the flour has been incorporated. This batter is thick, and as it sits, it gets a bit thicker.

5. Heat a 12- or 14-inch non-stick skillet or griddle over medium heat. Use a pastry brush to lightly coat the skillet with a tiny bit of oil, saving the rest for the remaining batches.

6. Scoop ¼ cup of the batter into the skillet to form a 4-inch griddle cake, using the back of a metal spoon to spread out the batter, if necessary. Reduce heat to medium-low. I fry three griddle cakes in one skillet.

7. The griddle cakes will be ready to flip when the undersides are a deep golden brown and the edges look cooked, 3 to 4 minutes.

8. Flip and cook for 3 to 5 more minutes, until the undersides are the same deep golden brown and the centres spring back when pressed. Place the cooked griddle cakes on the baking sheet and keep warm in the oven until you have cooked all 18 of them. Serve with pure maple syrup.

1 SERVING = 3 GRIDDLE CAKES WITHOUT MAPLE SYRUP
PER SERVING = 262 CALORIES, 7.6 G TOTAL FAT, 1.2 G SATURATED FAT, 0 G TRANS FAT, 64 MG CHOLESTEROL, 256 MG SODIUM, 34.8 G CARBOHYDRATE, 7.1 G FIBRE, 8.8 G SUGARS, 6 G ADDED SUGARS, 10.9 G PROTEIN, 436 MG POTASSIUM
CARBOHYDRATE CHOICE = 2 CHOICES

Weekend Pancakes for a Crowd VEG · *Serves 9*

WHEN I BEGAN WRITING THIS COOKBOOK, I knew I wanted a recipe that you could feed to a pack of hungry teenagers after a sleepover, to a crowd at a cottage, or to friends as a brunch item. I experimented so many times that my husband finally asked me to make the kitchen a pancake-free zone for a while, as he'd reached his pinnacle of pancake pigging out. I listened to him and took a much-needed pancake recipe-development hiatus. Several months later, I hit the kitchen armed with some new ideas, and here's what happened: lovely, not too dense, heart-healthy, colon-loving pancakes for the win! Totally worth the pancake moratorium, reminding me that sometimes listening to my husband is a very good idea.

WET INGREDIENTS

1 cup canned lentils, rinsed and well drained (see note on page 29)

½ cup oat bran

4 omega-3 eggs

3¼ cups skim milk, or soy or almond beverage

1 Tbsp pure vanilla extract

DRY INGREDIENTS

1½ cups whole grain barley flour

1 cup whole wheat flour

1 cup ground flaxseed (see page 184)

2 Tbsp natural wheat germ

2 Tbsp baking powder

2 Tbsp cinnamon

2 cups fresh (not frozen) local blueberries, rinsed and patted dry (optional)

2 Tbsp canola oil for the pancake griddle or frying pan (divided)

Pure amber maple syrup, for serving

1 SERVING = 3 PANCAKES WITHOUT BLUEBERRIES OR MAPLE SYRUP
PER SERVING: 306 CALORIES, 8.9 G TOTAL FAT, 1.4 G SATURATED FAT, 0 G TRANS FAT, 87 MG CHOLESTEROL, 342 MG SODIUM, 39.8 G CARBOHYDRATE, 10.3 G FIBRE, 5.6 G SUGARS, 0.2 G ADDED SUGARS, 14.9 G PROTEIN, 523 MG POTASSIUM
CARBOHYDRATE CHOICE = 2 CHOICES

1. Prepare the wet ingredients. Purée the lentils, oat bran, eggs, milk (or soy or almond beverage), and vanilla in a blender or in a large bowl using a hand-held immersion blender. Whirl until smooth. Let sit for 5 to 10 minutes.

2. Prepare the dry ingredients. In a large bowl, whisk together both flours, flaxseed, wheat germ, baking powder, and cinnamon.

3. Whirl up the wet ingredients again, pour into the dry ingredients, and whisk well. Gently fold in the blueberries, if using. Let the batter rest for 4 to 6 minutes in a pancake time-out.

4. While the batter is resting, preheat a pancake griddle to 350°F or heat a 12- or 14-inch non-stick skillet over medium heat. Preheat the oven to 200°F to keep the pancakes warm while you finish cooking. You do want to be eating with the whole gang, right? Place a cooling rack on top of a large rimmed baking sheet so the cooked pancakes don't steam in the oven while you finish the rest of them.

5. When the griddle or skillet is hot, stir the batter again. Use a pastry brush to lightly oil the griddle or pan, saving the rest of the oil for the remaining batches.

6. Scoop out ¼ cup of the batter and pour into the pan. Cook the pancakes for 3 to 5 minutes, flipping when the bottoms are a deep golden brown and bubbles appear on the top. Cook on the second side for 2 to 4 minutes, until the pancakes spring back when touched.

7. Place the cooked pancakes on the rack on the baking sheet and cover with a large piece of parchment paper or foil so they don't dry out. Keep them warm in the oven while you continue to cook the rest of the batter.

8. Serve with pure maple syrup if desired.

NOTE: Every so often, I stumble across a brilliant idea that I wish I'd come up with. When I was working on *Homegrown*, fellow PHEc Trevor Arsenault submitted a fabulous waffle recipe using red lentils. It was a stroke of genius, adding protein and fibre to a waffle, and left me wondering why I, the self-proclaimed Queen of Fibre, hadn't thought of that. Thanks for the inspiration, Trevor.

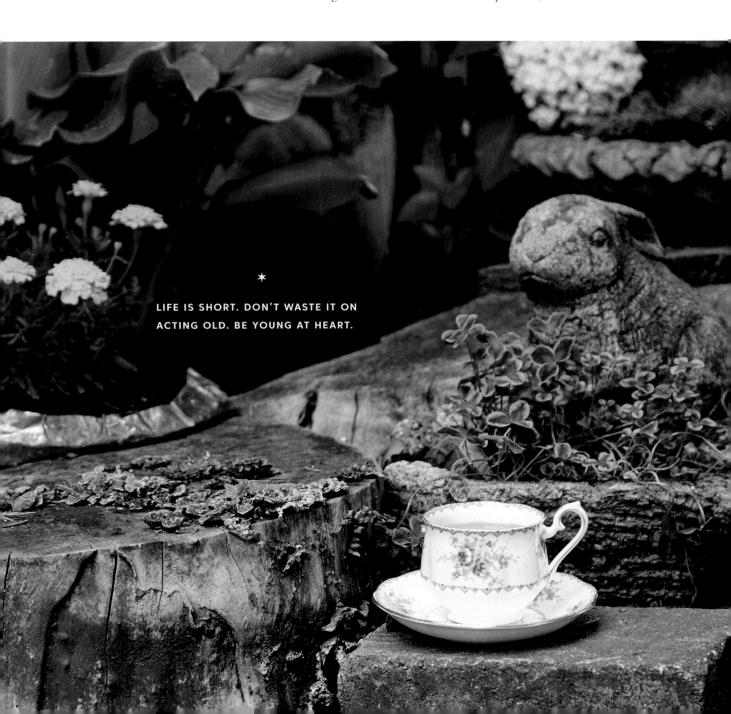

✳

LIFE IS SHORT. DON'T WASTE IT ON
ACTING OLD. BE YOUNG AT HEART.

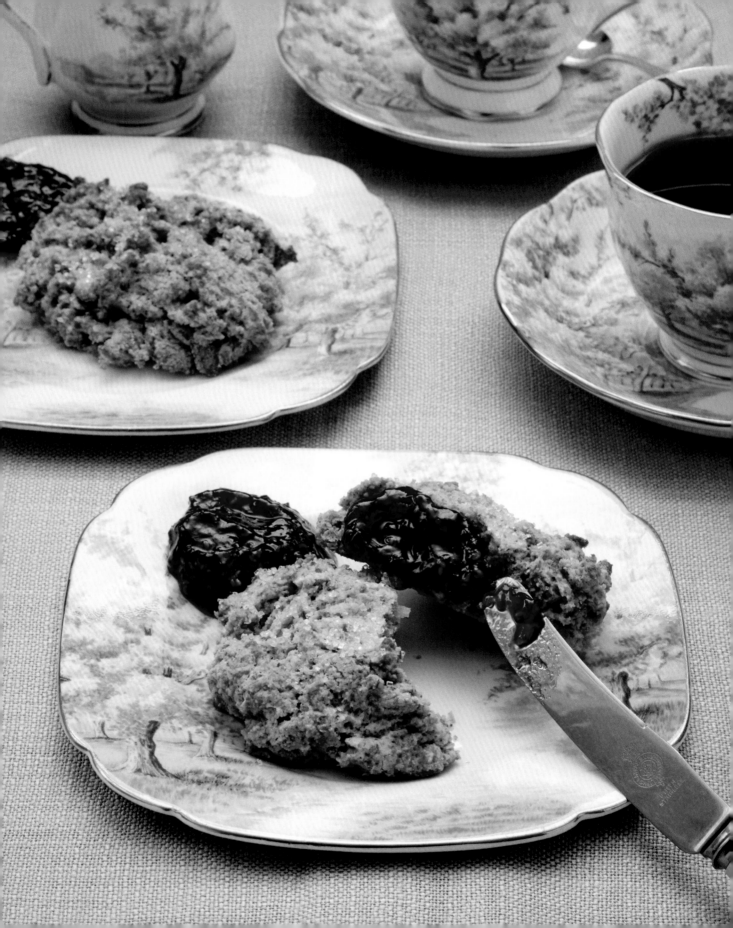

Ginger & Orange Drop Tea Biscuits VEG · *Makes 9 biscuits*

OH, ME ENGLISH, IRISH, AND SCOTTISH ROOTS ARE SHOWING HERE. Give me a tea biscuit and a proper cup of tea served in a china cup and saucer, and I'm pretty much your friend forever. Tea biscuits by their nature are empty calorie yum fests, but these, my fellow biscuit lovers, are fibre yum fests. Bake up a batch, put on the kettle, set out your good dishes, grab some jam, and enjoy.

1¼ cups whole grain barley flour

½ cup all-purpose flour

¼ cup flaxseed meal
(see page 184)

2 Tbsp granulated sugar

1 Tbsp baking powder

¼ tsp table salt

¼ cup cold unsalted butter,
cut in 1-inch cubes

2 Tbsp diced dried candied
ginger (see note on page 200)

1 Tbsp orange zest

½ cup skim milk

2 Tbsp canola oil

1 omega-3 egg

1 tsp coarse or sanding sugar

1. Place a rack in the middle of the oven and preheat the oven to 375°F. Line a rimless baking sheet with parchment paper. Set aside.

2. In a large bowl, whisk together the barley flour, all-purpose flour, flaxseed meal, sugar, baking powder, and salt.

3. Using a pastry blender or two knives, cut in the butter until it looks pea-sized. Using a fork, stir in the candied ginger and orange zest, making sure they are well distributed.

4. In a small bowl or a 1-cup glass measuring cup, whisk together the milk, oil, and egg. Pour the mixture into the dry ingredients and, using a rubber spatula, gently stir until the mixture doesn't have any visible dry flour. It will be sticky.

5. Using two tablespoons (the ones in your cutlery drawer), spoon out 9 equal portions, about a heaping ¼ cup each, onto the prepared baking sheet. Sprinkle each biscuit with a pinch of the coarse sugar.

6. Bake for 16 to 18 minutes. When they're ready, they will have flecks of golden brown on top. Remove the biscuits from the oven and place individually on a wire cooling rack. Serve warm or at room temperature with a dollop of raspberry jam.

1 SERVING = 1 BISCUIT
PER SERVING: 214 CALORIES, 10.4 G TOTAL FAT, 3.8 G SATURATED FAT, 0 G TRANS FAT, 23 MG CHOLESTEROL, 206 MG SODIUM, 25.5 G CARBOHYDRATE, 3.8 G FIBRE, 7.4 G SUGARS, 4.9 G ADDED SUGARS, 4.4 G PROTEIN, 163 MG POTASSIUM
CARBOHYDRATE CHOICE = 1½ CHOICES

Spring Quiche VEG GF · *Serves 6*

QUICHE WAS ALL THE RAGE BACK IN THE LATE '70S. Every brunch I attended for about seven years had at least one quiche. I was quiched-out by the early '80s and I vowed I'd never eat another piece again, until I tried fellow PHEc Erica Horner's recipe. It was goodbye to the heavy pastry crust that always ended up soggy, adieu to all the saturated fat, and hello to a quinoa crust. Here's my higher-fibre version of Erica's quinoa crust, with an egg custard filling that is an homage to spring flavours. Serve this for dinner or as a brunch item.

8 oz (225 g) fresh local asparagus

QUICHE CRUST

½ cup quinoa

¼ cup flaxseed meal (see page 184)

¼ cup pasteurized egg whites (see note on page 49)

FILLING

6 omega-3 eggs

¼ cup pasteurized egg whites

1 Tbsp grainy Dijon mustard

½ tsp dry mustard

¼ tsp freshly ground black pepper

⅛ tsp table salt

1 (5 oz/140 g) package low-fat or reduced-fat goat cheese

3 green onions, whites included, thinly sliced

¼ cup + 2 Tbsp finely chopped fresh dill

1. Rinse the asparagus and either snap off the woody stalks or cut them off. Cut the asparagus into ¼- or ½-inch pieces, depending on the thickness of the stalks. Skinny stalks should be cut into ½-inch pieces, and thicker stalks should be cut into ¼-inch pieces. Make sure to keep the tops intact. Separate the tops from the stalks and reserve the tops.

2. To make the quiche crust, rinse the quinoa in a fine-mesh strainer. Tip into a small 1½-quart saucepan—the size is important here. Add 1 cup water and bring to a boil. Cover, reduce heat to a low simmer (it should be bubbling but not boiling), and cook for 10 to 14 minutes.

3. Meanwhile, in a medium bowl, whisk together the flaxseed meal and egg whites and set aside while the quinoa cooks. This is a really important step. The flaxseed meal needs to absorb some of the egg whites before you add the cooked quinoa.

4. The quinoa is done when the grains are translucent and all the water has been absorbed. Fluff with a fork, remove from heat, and let stand for 5 to 10 minutes.

5. Preheat the oven to 400°F. Line a 10-inch metal pie plate with wet parchment paper (see page 15). Shape the parchment into the pie plate; the paper should be as malleable as pastry dough. Trim the top so there is about a ½-inch overhang. Set aside.

6. Make the filling. In a medium bowl, whisk together the eggs and egg whites. Add the Dijon, dry mustard, pepper, and salt, then set aside. Have the goat cheese, green onions, and dill ready to go.

7. By now, the quinoa should be fluffy and ready to add to the flaxseed mixture from Step 3. Mix together well, then tip into the prepared pie plate. Using the back of a metal tablespoon, push the mixture from the bottom of the pan up the sides, right to the top of the pie plate. You want to evenly cover the pan with a thin layer of the quinoa mixture.

recipe continues

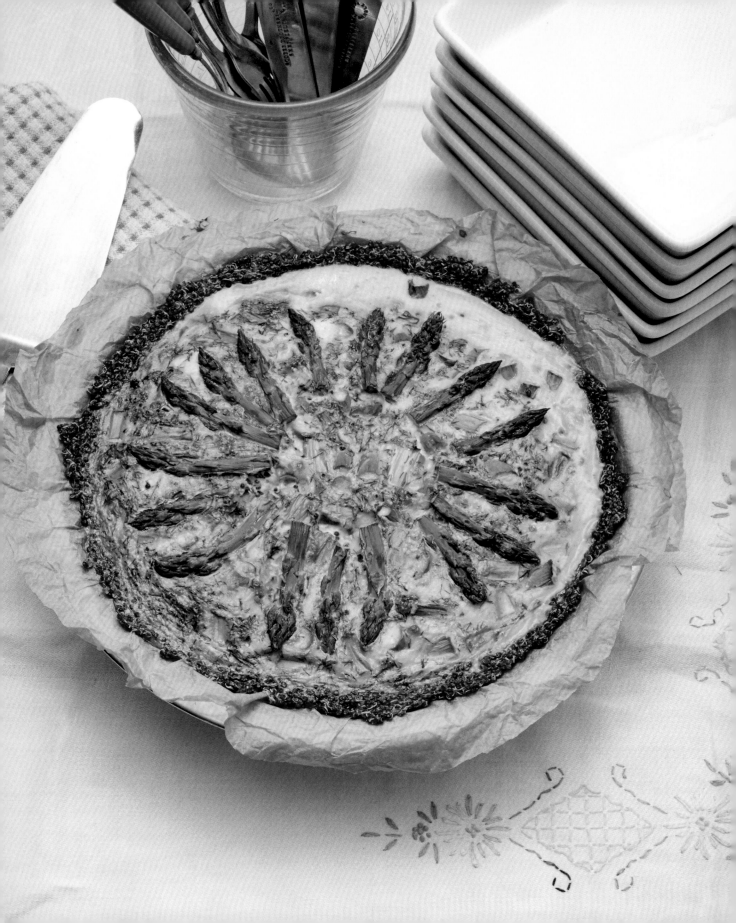

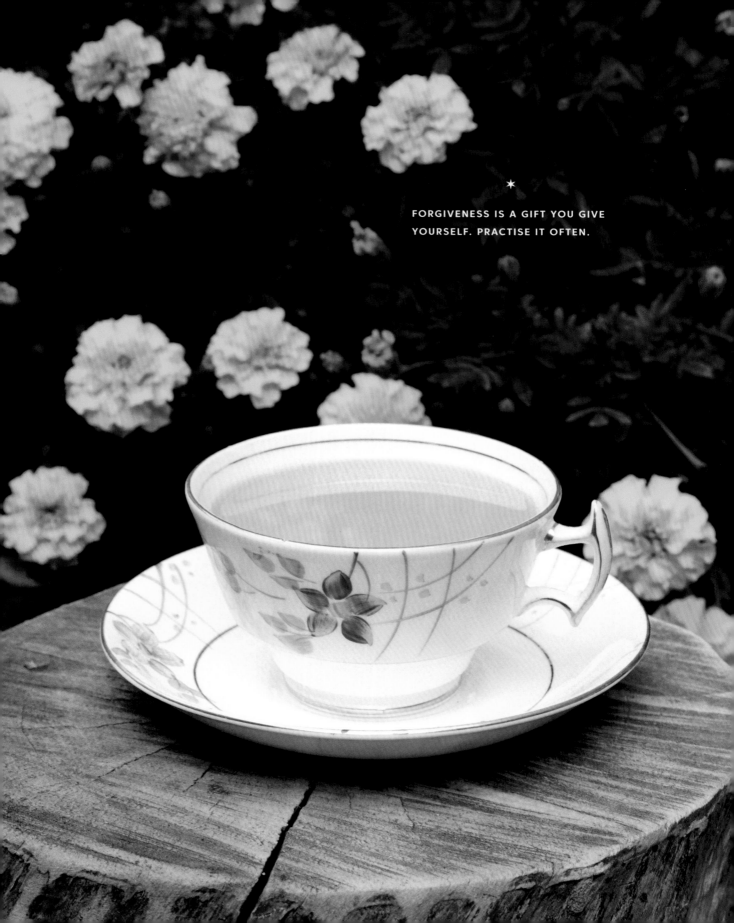

FORGIVENESS IS A GIFT YOU GIVE
YOURSELF. PRACTISE IT OFTEN.

NOTE: Pasteurized egg whites can be found with the whole eggs in your local grocery store. They are sold in cartons. Once the carton is opened, you need to use up the egg whites within 7 days. Feel free to use fresh egg whites in this recipe if desired.

8. Assemble the quiche. Evenly crumble the goat cheese so that it covers the bottom of the crust, followed by the green onions and dill. Add the asparagus, except for the reserved tips.

9. Pour the egg mixture over the crust, then place the asparagus tips on top. The accompanying photograph (page 47) shows what my husband did (yes, he helped during the photo shoots), or go rogue and do your own thing.

10. Bake for 55 to 60 minutes or until the centre is firm and a toothpick inserted in the centre comes out clean.

11. Remove the quiche from the oven and let it sit for at least 5 minutes and up to 30 minutes before slicing. Gently lift the quiche from the pan, holding onto the parchment paper. Place on a cutting board and cut into six equal pieces. Leftovers can be stored in the fridge for up to 2 days, and they taste great cold.

1 SERVING = ⅙ OF THE QUICHE
PER SERVING: 239 CALORIES, 13.3 G TOTAL FAT, 5.3 G SATURATED FAT, 0 G TRANS FAT, 203 MG CHOLESTEROL, 264 MG SODIUM, 13.7 G CARBOHYDRATE, 3.3 G FIBRE, 1.9 G SUGARS, 0 G ADDED SUGARS, 15.8 G PROTEIN, 307 MG POTASSIUM
CARBOHYDRATE CHOICE = ½ CHOICE

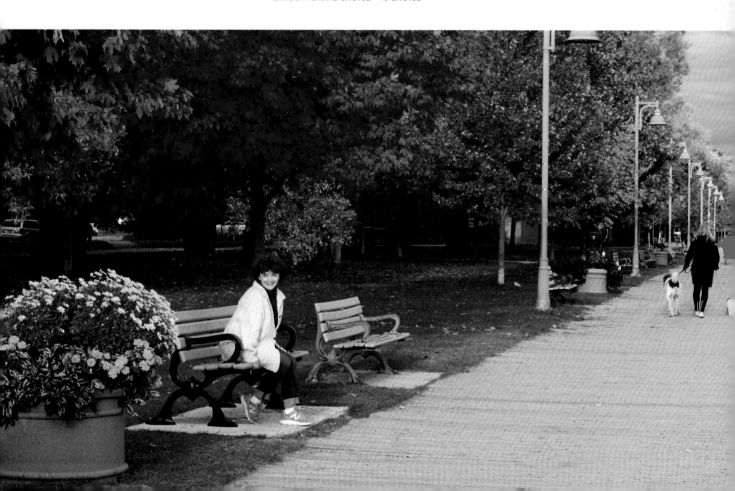

Morning Eggs Mexican-Style VEG GF · *Serves 2*

WHEN I WAS PREGNANT WITH MY SON, I craved eggs and beans so much that I ate them for breakfast almost every day for six months, complete with freshly ground black pepper and tons of hot sauce. After my son was born, all I seemed to have time for was a spoonful of peanut butter and a huge glass of orange juice in the morning. The eggs and beans became a distant memory. Fast-forward many years and enter Pinterest. I was lying in a heap on my couch browsing the food sites when I happened to see one lone picture of eggs and beans. It tweaked a food memory and got me off the couch and into my kitchen. Apparently, you don't have to be pregnant to love this.

1 tsp canola oil

1 small zucchini or ½ medium zucchini, diced

2 cups grape tomatoes, halved (about 20)

1¼ cups canned no-salt-added black beans, rinsed and well drained (see note)

2 omega-3 eggs

½ cup (2 oz/56 g) grated old Cheddar cheese

1 green onion, whites included, finely chopped

Hot sauce, for serving (optional)

NOTE: Save the extra canned beans in a covered container in the fridge and add them to salads or soups for a hit of protein and fibre.

1. Heat a 12- or 14-inch non-stick skillet over medium heat, and add the oil. If you're using a cast-iron pan, you will need to add a bit more oil. Toss in the zucchini and sauté for 1 to 2 minutes, until it starts to soften. Add the tomatoes and sauté for another minute. Stir in the black beans.

2. Using a wooden spoon or a heat-safe spatula, make two shallow indentations in the vegetable/bean mixture, then crack an egg into each opening. It's going to look like two eyes staring at you, in a good way.

3. Cover the pan with a lid, reduce heat to low, and cook the eggs until your desired yolk doneness. I like mine sort of runny with a big hit of egg yolk ooze, which takes 3 to 4 minutes.

4. Remove the skillet from the heat, sprinkle with the cheese and green onion, cover, and let the cheese melt.

5. To serve, divide the mixture in half and gently transfer the egg and the vegetables to a shallow bowl or a plate. Add hot sauce if desired.

1 SERVING = ½ OF THE RECIPE
PER SERVING: 421 CALORIES, 19.6 G TOTAL FAT, 7.8 G SATURATED FAT, 0 G TRANS FAT, 223 MG CHOLESTEROL, 276 MG SODIUM, 38.3 G CARBOHYDRATE, 10.2 G FIBRE, 7.5 G SUGARS, 0 G ADDED SUGARS, 26.9 G PROTEIN, 1117 MG POTASSIUM
CARBOHYDRATE CHOICE = 2 CHOICES

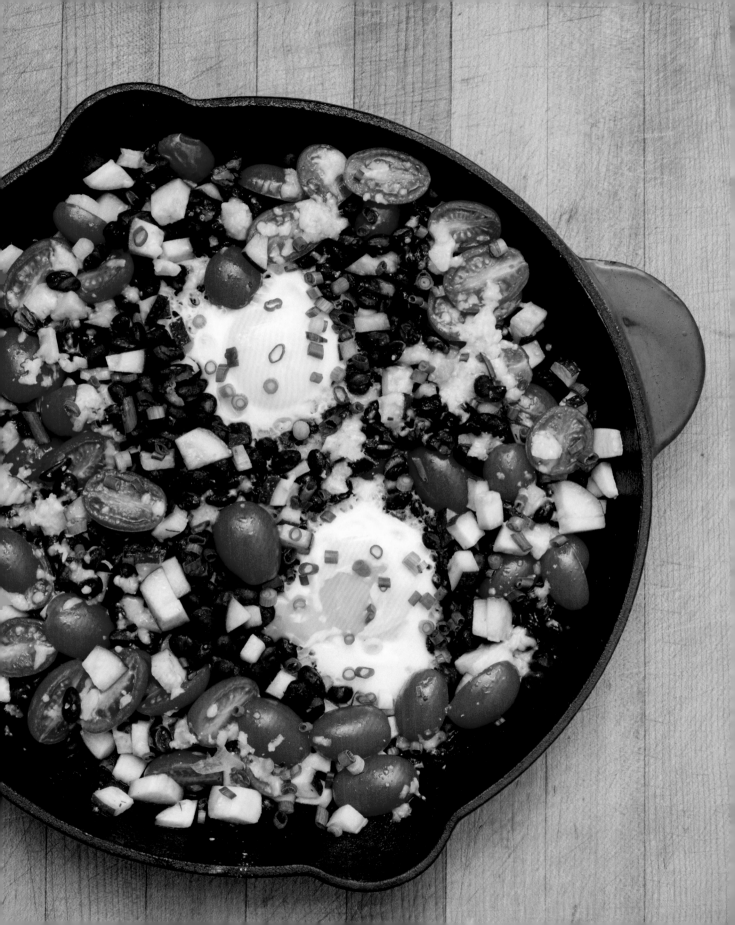

Mairlyn's Energy Balls   VEG · *Makes 34 balls*

WHILE I WAS CREATING MY FIBRE-RICH RECIPE FOR ENERGY BALLS, I decided to add psyllium (a.k.a. nature's blasting gel), without realizing that it swells up and can get stuck in your throat. The energy ball I popped into my mouth got stuck somewhere between my breast bone and the tube leading into my stomach. Three giant glasses of water later, I was bloated and felt like I might die. My Girl Guide brain turned on and I decided I should jump off a chair, rationalizing that gravity and the swift jerking motion when I hit the ground would cause the ball of quick-forming cement to move its way into my gut. That sort of worked. I was all alone, so I called my BFF in California to see if she had any great ideas. She suggested a hot bath and deep breathing. All I could think was "my kingdom for an Ativan." It took about five hours to feel normal. By then I was a wrinkled-up prune with wicked gas, but alive. Please learn from my mistake: never add psyllium to a raw energy ball. I'm filing this debacle under the perils of recipe developing.

1½ cups large oat flakes

½ cup dark or bittersweet chocolate chips

¼ cup natural cocoa powder

½ cup ground flaxseed (see page 184)

½ cup oat bran

1 cup natural almond or peanut butter

½ cup molasses or liquid honey

2 Tbsp pure vanilla extract

NOTE: For kids under five years old, one serving = one energy ball. Do not serve to children under three years old.

1. In the bowl of a food processor fitted with the steel blade attachment, pulse the oats and chocolate chips. It's going to be noisy, but pulse until the chocolate chips look like smaller bits of chocolate, about 1 minute.

2. Add the cocoa powder and pulse again. Add the flaxseed and oat bran and pulse until the ingredients are well distributed. Add the almond or peanut butter, molasses or honey, and vanilla and pulse until it all comes together in a giant ball.

3. Form the mixture into 34 equally sized balls, using your hands to form each one. The heat from your hands will help them stick together. If you're measuring, use about 1 Tbsp of the mixture per ball.

4. Line a container with a tight-fitting lid with parchment paper, and place a layer of energy balls over top. Place a second layer of parchment paper over the energy balls and continue. Store in the fridge for up to 1 week.

1 SERVING = 3 BALLS
PER SERVING: 345 CALORIES, 18.8 G TOTAL FAT, 2.5 G SATURATED FAT, 0 G TRANS FAT, 0 MG CHOLESTEROL, 10 MG SODIUM, 39.8 G CARBOHYDRATE, 7.6 G FIBRE, 16.2 G SUGARS, 15 G ADDED SUGARS, 11.4 G PROTEIN, 612 MG POTASSIUM
CARBOHYDRATE CHOICE = 2½ CHOICES

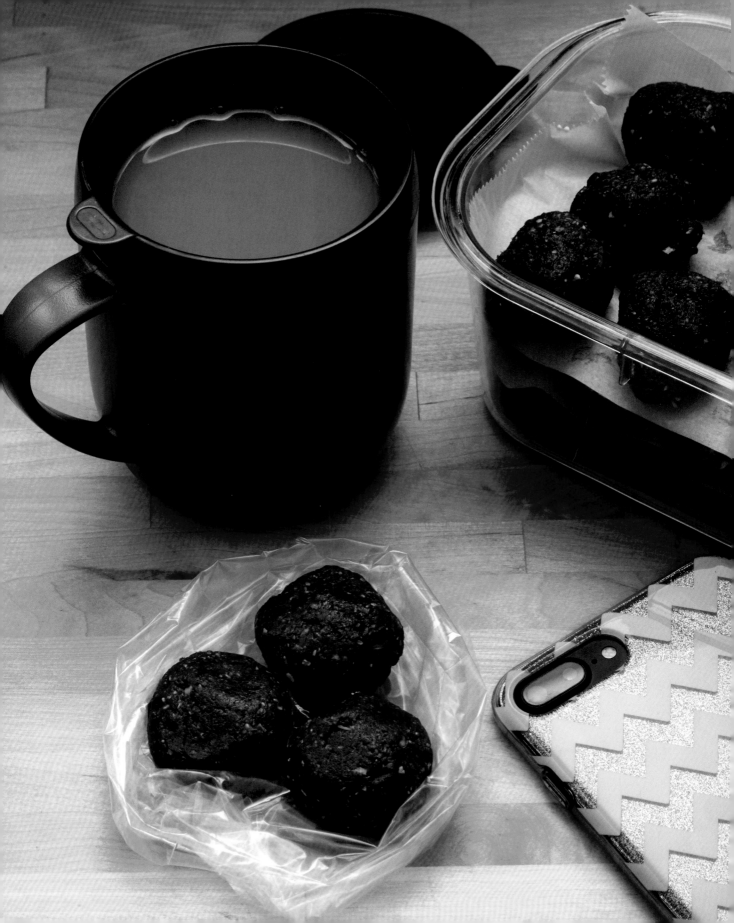

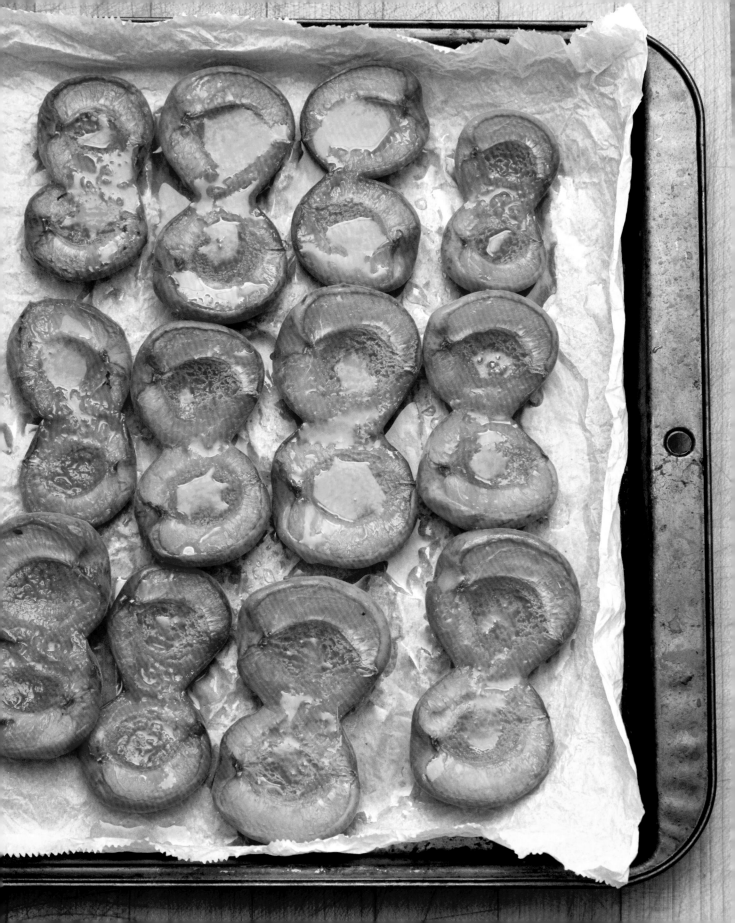

Honey-Roasted Apricots VEG LF GF · *Makes 6 cups*

THE DAY I CAME UP WITH THE IDEA TO MAKE HONEY-ROASTED APRICOTS, it was hot, hazy, and humid. I had a ton of apricots and I was planning on making apricot jam, but adding more humidity to my house seemed insane. To avoid the humid heat from jam making, I decided to oven-roast them instead. I was talking to my BFF Michale on the phone when the timer went off. I managed to get them out of the oven and still talk to her on the phone. (First red flag of impending doom.) They were so gorgeous, I thought, why not head out to the front porch, take a picture of them, and send it to her while we were talking? Cradling the phone with my ear and shoulder, I carried the pan through the living room, and as I tried to open the front screen door, disaster hit. I dropped the entire pan, face down, on my front-door welcome mat. I think my explosive superlatives are still floating somewhere in space. Not only did I have to throw out the entire pan of golden deliciousness, but I had to basically hose down my front porch so there wouldn't be a racoon convention there that night. Moral of the story: I need an assistant.

3 lb (1.4 kg) whole, medium-ripe apricots (about 28)

¾ cup liquid honey

1. Preheat the oven to 250°F and line a large rimmed baking sheet with wet parchment paper (see page 15).

2. Rinse the apricots, pat them dry, and cut off any bruises. Cut or pull the apricots into halves and remove and discard the pits.

3. Place the apricot halves peel side down on the prepared baking sheet. Drizzle with the honey. Roast in the oven for about 2 hours, until they turn deep golden. Remove and let sit for 5 minutes.

4. Transfer the apricots to the bowl of a food processor fitted with the steel blade attachment and purée until smooth or, if you prefer, slightly chunky. They are very soft, so this step happens quickly.

5. Freeze in ¼- or ½-cup portions. Use 2 Tbsp as a topping for yogurt, ½ cup over Camembert, or as an ingredient in a chicken or pork dish.

1 SERVING = 2 TBSP
PER SERVING: 25 CALORIES, 0.1 G TOTAL FAT, 0 G SATURATED FAT, 0 G TRANS FAT,
0 MG CHOLESTEROL, 0 MG SODIUM, 6.4 G CARBOHYDRATE, 0.4 G FIBRE, 6 G SUGARS,
4.2 G ADDED SUGARS, 0.3 G PROTEIN, 53 MG POTASSIUM
CARBOHYDRATE CHOICE = < 1 CHOICE

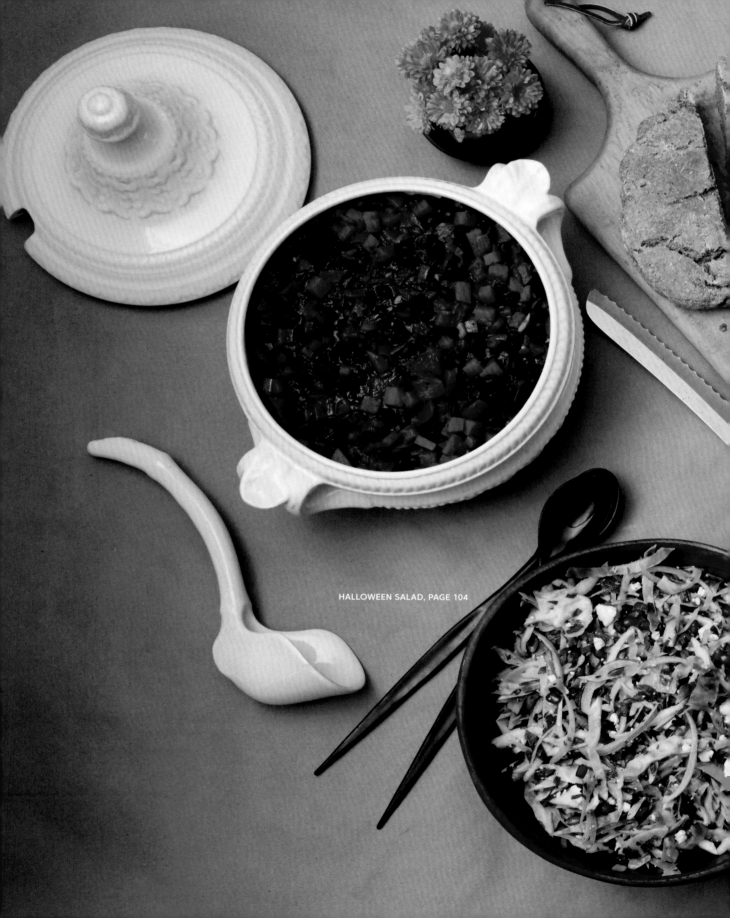

HALLOWEEN SALAD, PAGE 104

IRISH SODA BREAD, PAGE 75

Soups
&
Dinner
Breads

SPLIT PEA SOUP WITH
SMOKED HAM, PAGE 69

Soups can be made any time of year, but I prefer fall and winter soups to the lighter spring and summer soups. I like the stick-to-your-ribs soups that become dinner in a bowl. When the nights start getting colder and fall vegetables hit the farmers' market, I get out my soup pot.

Stock vs. Broth

The main difference between stock and broth is that stock has a much bolder flavour than broth. Broth is a one-note pony. It's a clear liquid made by boiling one protein (meat, fish, or poultry, all with fresh bones) with water or just vegetables with water. You can buy broth in cans, in Tetra Paks, or in a dried version either as a powder or a cube.

Stock is a versatile cornucopia of flavours. It's made by slowly simmering one protein (meat, fish, or poultry with fresh bones as well as the meat) with water and added vegetables and seasonings. You can make your own stock and save money on your grocery bill by reserving the ends of the vegetables you use in your daily cooking and adding a protein source with bones as well as seasonings. Or you can buy it at a higher-end grocery store.

I use broth in the recipes in this book because it's an easier and more accessible choice for most people. If you have homemade stock, use it instead of the broth for a heartier flavour in all the soups. If you make your own stock, don't add any salt. Use the amount listed in the recipe. If you buy stock with salt, eliminate the salt in the recipe.

One of my favourite ways to entertain in the fall and winter months is to throw a soup party. I always serve two soups, plus bread and a salad. It's easy and fun, and if you use brown butcher paper instead of a tablecloth, you can write what everything is right on the paper.

To throw a soup party for six to eight people, try the following:

- Split Pea Soup with Smoked Ham (page 69)
- Irish Soda Bread (page 75)
- Halloween Salad (page 104)
- Wine (optional . . . as if!)

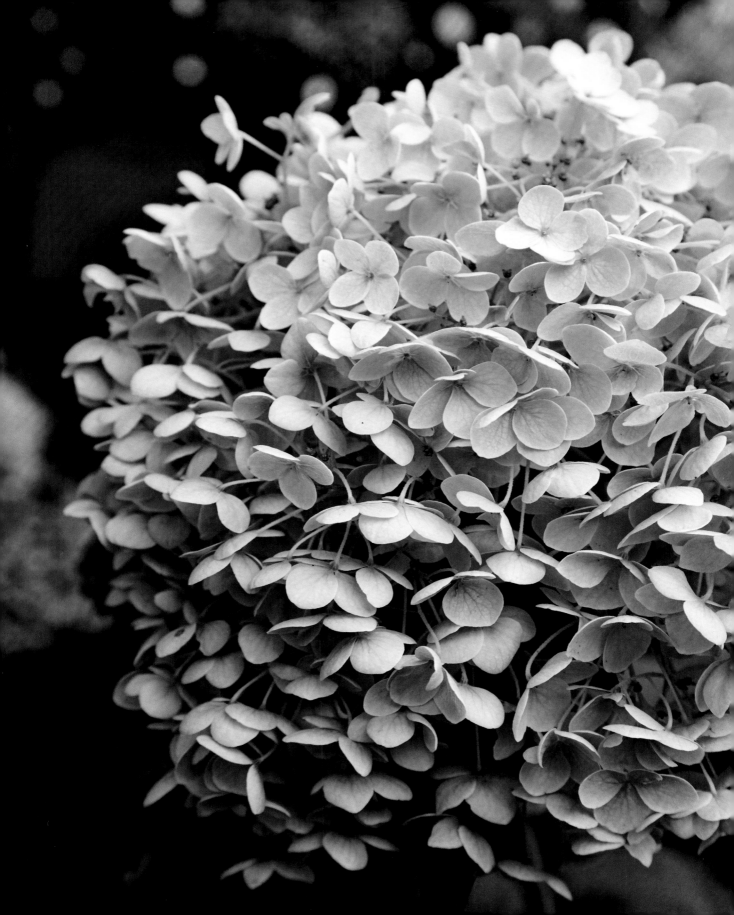

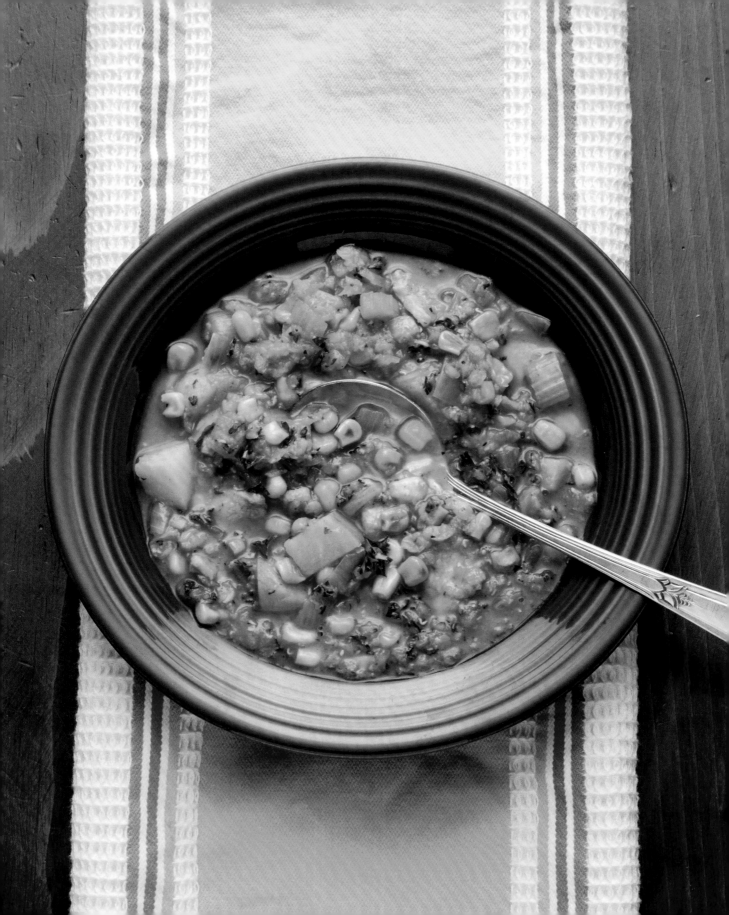

Grilled Corn Chowder LF · *Serves 8*

I LOVE MY FARMERS' MARKET BECAUSE I LOVE TO DECIDE what to make for dinner on a given week based on what foods are ripe and ready. When the last of the local corn on the cob is in season, I make this soup as an homage to my local corn. Grilling the corn brings out its natural sweetness and adds a smoky note.

2 Tbsp canola oil

5 slices (about 8 oz/225 g) back bacon or peameal bacon, cut in small pieces

2 onions, diced

1 medium yellow-fleshed potato, scrubbed well and diced in ½-inch cubes

1 stalk celery, diced

2 tsp smoked paprika

4 cups no-salt-added chicken broth

1 cup dried red lentils

1 tsp table salt

½ tsp freshly ground black pepper

4 cups grilled corn (about 4 cobs)

1 cup finely chopped fresh parsley, leaves and stems

NOTE: When it comes to my favourite F-word, fibre, soups are another way to add more vegetables and pulses, like lentils, to your diet, upping your fibre intake one spoonful at a time.

1. Heat a Dutch oven or a large saucepan over medium heat. Add the oil and bacon and sauté for 1 minute. Add the onions and sauté for 3 to 5 minutes, until the onions start to become soft. Add the potato, celery, and paprika and sauté for 1 minute.

2. Add the broth, lentils, salt, and pepper. Stir well, scraping any browned bits from the bottom of the pot to prevent burning and to add more fabulous flavour.

3. Bring the soup to a boil, cover, reduce heat to a simmer, and cook for 20 minutes, until the lentils are extremely soft. Add the corn and return to a boil, then cover, reduce heat to a simmer, and cook until the corn is heated through, 3 to 5 minutes.

4. Remove from heat, stir in the parsley, and serve.

1 SERVING = 1 CUP
PER SERVING: 295 CALORIES, 5.8 G TOTAL FAT, 0.8 G SATURATED FAT, 0 G TRANS FAT, 21 MG CHOLESTEROL, 560 MG SODIUM, 47.9 G CARBOHYDRATE, 5.8 G FIBRE, 6.2 G SUGARS, 0 G ADDED SUGARS, 16.9 G PROTEIN, 1014 MG POTASSIUM
CARBOHYDRATE CHOICE = 3 CHOICES

Fresh & Wild Mushroom Barley Soup VEG V LF · *Serves 4*

INSPIRED BY THE DREARY FALL AND THE WICKEDLY COLD WINTER WEATHER, this stick-to-your-ribs soup is so thick and flavourful that I wanted to call it a chowder. But the rules of soup naming prevailed, so it is technically a soup, albeit an extremely thick one.

2½ cups (2 oz/56 g) dried mixed wild mushrooms (see note on page 64)

2 cups boiling water

8 oz (225 g) fresh cremini mushrooms

2 Tbsp canola oil

8 cloves garlic, minced

2 onions, diced

2 tsp dried thyme leaves

¾ tsp freshly ground black pepper

¾ cup pot barley, rinsed

4 cups low-sodium mushroom broth (see note on page 64)

¼ cup chopped fresh parsley, leaves and stems

1. Rinse the dried mushrooms to make sure all dirt or grit is gone. You don't want crunchy particles in your soup. Place the mushrooms in a heat-safe 4-cup bowl or glass measuring cup.

2. Pour the boiling water over the dried mushrooms, cover, and let sit for 20 minutes. You are steeping the dried mushrooms to create an elixir of mushroom deliciousness.

3. While you are waiting for the dried mushrooms to be ready, gently rinse or wipe the cremini mushrooms with a damp paper towel to get rid of any dirt. Slice thinly.

4. Heat a Dutch oven or a large saucepan over medium heat, then add the oil and the cremini mushrooms, and leave them alone. Don't be bumping the mushrooms—you want to develop flavour by allowing them to brown. Depending on the size of your pot, this can take anywhere from 4 to 8 minutes. Sautéing or bumping them around encourages the water to leave the mushrooms and you end up with steamed mushrooms, which is not what you want in this recipe.

5. When the mushrooms have browned, add the garlic and onions and sauté for 1 minute. Add the thyme and pepper. Sauté until the onions have softened and have started to turn golden.

6. Huge tip: Place a fine-mesh strainer over a medium bowl. Gently pour the soaking dried mushrooms into the strainer; go slowly so that any dirt you may have missed in Step 1, which will have sunk to the bottom of the heat-safe bowl or measuring cup, stays behind. Remove the strainer. The liquid that is left over in the bottom bowl is the elixir of mushroom deliciousness. Set aside.

7. Coarsely chop the hydrated dried mushrooms, add them to the pot, and stir well. Pour in the mushroom broth and the elixir of mushroom deliciousness. Add the barley, then use the flat edge of a wooden spoon to scrape up any browned bits from the bottom of the pot.

recipe continues

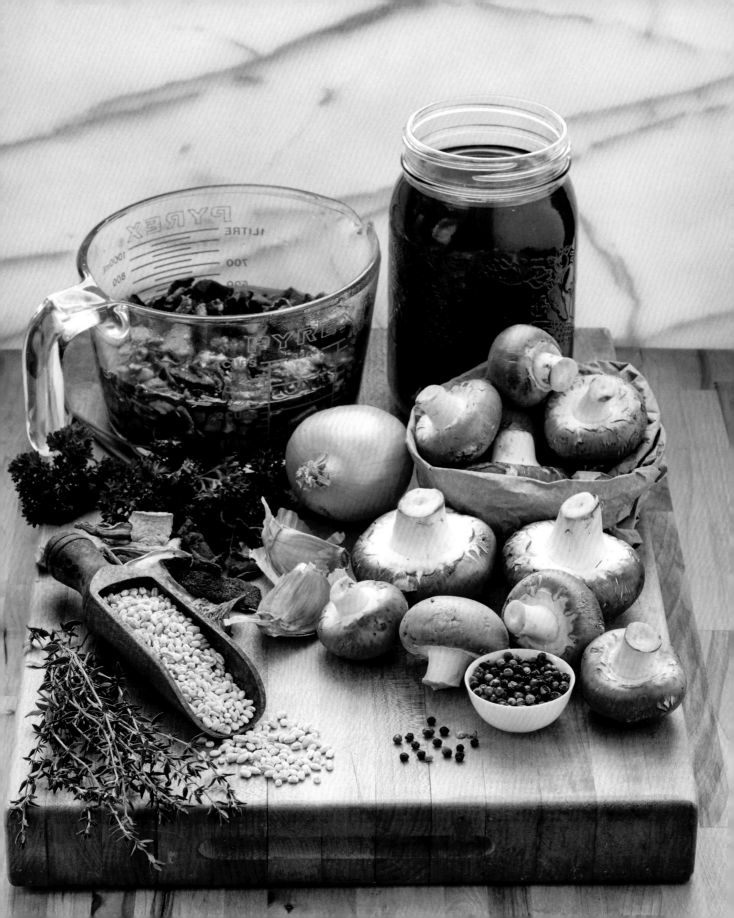

NOTE: You can find ready-to-use mushroom broth in the soup aisle in a Tetra Pak or in dried cubes. Look for one that has a lower sodium content (400 to 460 mg per 1-cup serving).

8. Cover the pot and bring it to a boil. Stir well, reduce heat to a simmer, and cover. Cook for 25 to 35 minutes, until the barley is soft but not mushy.

9. You now have a choice: to purée or not to purée? I like the texture of the whole mushrooms, but I also want the soup to be slightly puréed, so I gently use a hand-held immersion blender.

10. Divide the soup equally among four bowls and sprinkle each with 1 Tbsp chopped parsley.

1 SERVING = ABOUT 1½ CUPS
PER SERVING: 232 CALORIES, 8.2 G TOTAL FAT, 0.8 G SATURATED FAT, 0 G TRANS FAT,
0 MG CHOLESTEROL, 473 MG SODIUM, 35.9 G CARBOHYDRATE, 7.9 G FIBRE, 3.1 G SUGARS,
0 G ADDED SUGARS, 9.2 G PROTEIN, 561 MG POTASSIUM
CARBOHYDRATE CHOICE = 2 CHOICES

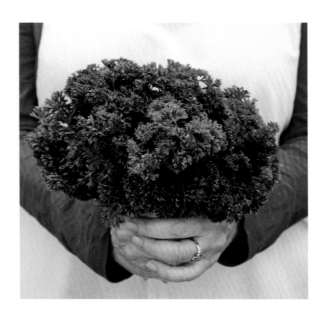

Asian-Style Vegetable Soup with Soba Noodles LF · *Serves 4*

THIS MAIN-COURSE ENTRÉE IS MORE LIKE A NOODLE DISH with vegetables and broth than a true soup. It's easy to make if you prep everything before you start cooking, because once it starts, it's bingo, bango, boom and dinner's ready.

½ medium sweet potato

1 heaping cup (about 4½ oz/ 125 g) snow peas

3 baby bok choy

1 (5.3 oz/150 g) package enoki mushrooms

1 (12 oz/350 g) package extra-firm tofu

4 cups no-salt-added chicken broth or vegetable broth

2 bundles (about 6½ oz/185 g) buckwheat soba noodles (see note on page 66)

1 Tbsp red miso paste

3 Tbsp lower-sodium or lite tamari

6 cloves garlic, minced

2-inch piece fresh ginger, julienned (about 3 Tbsp)

1. Fill a large saucepan three-quarters full of cold water and bring to a boil over high heat.

2. Meanwhile, prep all vegetables. Peel the sweet potato, cut in half lengthwise, then cut into ¼-inch half moons. Set aside.

3. Rinse the snow peas and bok choy. Cut the ends off the snow peas and leave whole. Cut off the ends of the bok choy and slice into ½-inch pieces. Set aside.

4. Cut the enoki mushrooms away from the base. You want them to be individual pieces, not one lump. Save the base for your next stir-fry or stock recipe, but remember to use it within 2 to 3 days.

5. Remove the tofu from the package and drain any liquid. Cut into ½-inch cubes and set aside.

6. Once you finish the vegetable and tofu prep, pour the chicken or vegetable broth into a large saucepan or a Dutch oven and bring to a boil. The pot of water from Step 1 should be boiling by now (it's all about timing in this recipe).

7. Add the noodles to the boiling water, return to a gentle boil, and gently stir to make sure they aren't all stuck together. Reduce heat to a simmer and cook, uncovered, for 3 minutes, until the noodles are tender (or cook according to the manufacturer's directions). DON'T OVERCOOK THESE—sorry, was I yelling? They go from tender to a lump of mush quickly. Drain the noodles and lightly rinse with cold water. Leave the noodles in the strainer.

8. By now the chicken or vegetable broth should be boiling. Add the sweet potato, cover the pot, reduce heat to a simmer, and cook for 2 minutes. Add the tofu and continue to cook until the sweet potato is slightly soft. Add the miso paste, tamari, garlic, and ginger and stir well.

recipe continues

NOTE: Buckwheat soba noodles are usually made with 100% buckwheat flour, which is gluten-free and very delicate. You can find soba noodles in the Asian food section of the grocery store. Within the package, the noodles are often wrapped in smaller bundles, but if you've bought noodles that don't come in bundles, the equivalent to two bundles is about 6½ oz (185 g), or two handfuls.

9. Remove the soup from the heat and add the snow peas, bok choy, and mushrooms. Gently stir, cover, and let sit while you divide the noodles equally among four deep Asian-style soup bowls.

10. Stir the soup once more to evenly distribute the vegetables. Using a slotted spoon, scoop out the vegetables and tofu and place them on top of the noodles. Try to make sure every bowl is getting an equal amount of vegetables and tofu. Divide the remaining broth equally among the bowls and serve. I like to use chopsticks and an Asian-style soup spoon to eat this.

1 SERVING = ¼ OF THE RECIPE
PER SERVING: 291 CALORIES, 2.5 G TOTAL FAT, 0.3 G SATURATED FAT, 0 G TRANS FAT, 0 MG CHOLESTEROL, 1237 MG SODIUM, 53.6 G CARBOHYDRATE, 3.2 G FIBRE, 5.4 G SUGARS, 0 G ADDED SUGARS, 16.9 G PROTEIN, 674 MG POTASSIUM
CARBOHYDRATE CHOICE = 3½ CHOICES

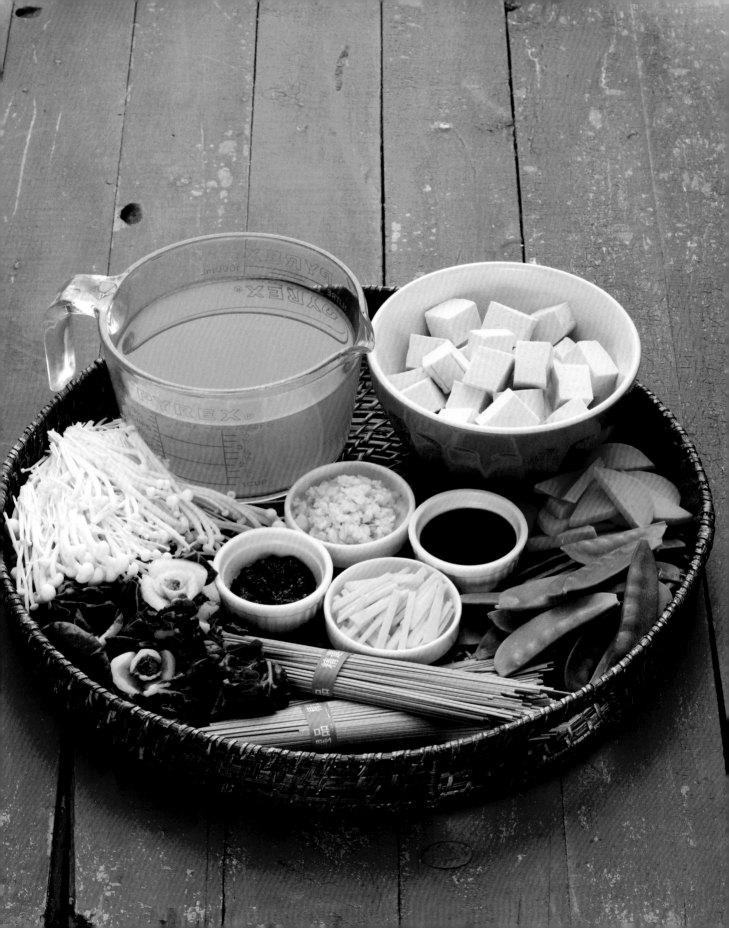

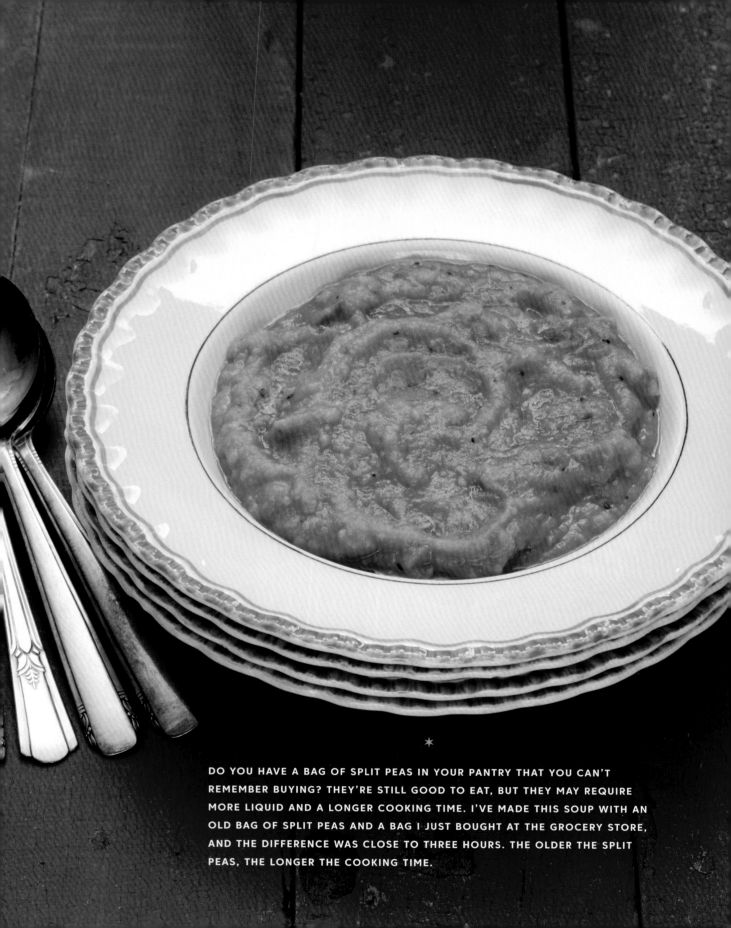

*

DO YOU HAVE A BAG OF SPLIT PEAS IN YOUR PANTRY THAT YOU CAN'T REMEMBER BUYING? THEY'RE STILL GOOD TO EAT, BUT THEY MAY REQUIRE MORE LIQUID AND A LONGER COOKING TIME. I'VE MADE THIS SOUP WITH AN OLD BAG OF SPLIT PEAS AND A BAG I JUST BOUGHT AT THE GROCERY STORE, AND THE DIFFERENCE WAS CLOSE TO THREE HOURS. THE OLDER THE SPLIT PEAS, THE LONGER THE COOKING TIME.

Split Pea Soup with Smoked Ham LF · *Serves 10 to 12*

I LOVE THE POWER OF FOOD MEMORIES. One whiff of pea soup and my soul is transported back in time to my parents' kitchen. My mom and dad are chopping onions and carrots, there is an enormous ham simmering in a gigantic soup pot, the windows are steamed up, and my forever-optimist father is excited about the prospect of his favourite soup for dinner. My parents were big into pea soup, and their perception was that a bowl of split pea soup had healing powers. Some kids got chicken soup when they were sick, but we got split pea soup so thick that a spoon could stand upright unaided by any mechanical devices. You could almost eat it with a fork. This is my tribute to that food memory and to my parents. They would be proud; my soup is just as thick as theirs.

8 cups no-salt-added chicken broth

6 large carrots, thinly sliced

3 onions, diced

4 cups yellow split peas, rinsed and well drained (see sidebar)

1¾ lb (800 g) fully cooked, smoked sodium-reduced ham, cut in ½-inch cubes (see note)

1 tsp freshly ground black pepper

NOTE: Some brands of ham use celery extract instead of nitrates. Celery has naturally occurring nitrates. If you are concerned about using smoked or cured products that include nitrates, look for a smoked ham that says "naturally smoked" or has celery extract in the list of ingredients. They are usually sold in smaller portions. Don't worry if there is less ham, as it will still infuse the soup with fabulous flavour.

1. Pour the chicken broth into a large soup pot. Add the carrots and onions and bring to a boil.

2. Add the split peas, ham, and pepper and bring the soup back to a boil. Stir well, cover, reduce heat to a simmer, and cook, stirring occasionally, for 1 to 1½ hours, until the split peas have softened completely. Divide into bowls and serve.

3. Freeze any leftover soup for a quick and easy family dinner, or freeze in smaller portions for a quick lunch. This already thick soup thickens even more in the fridge, so feel free to add some water when you reheat it.

1 SERVING = 1½ CUPS
PER SERVING: 391 CALORIES, 3.8 G TOTAL FAT, 1.5 G SATURATED FAT, 0 G TRANS FAT, 35 MG CHOLESTEROL, 605 MG SODIUM, 57.4 G CARBOHYDRATE, 6.8 G FIBRE, 9.5 G SUGARS, 1.4 G ADDED SUGARS, 32 G PROTEIN, 2006 MG POTASSIUM
CARBOHYDRATE COUNT = 3½ CHOICES

Tuscan White Bean Soup GF · *Serves 6*

THIS HEARTY SOUP IS A PERFECT DINNER FOR THOSE COLD, RAINY OR SNOWY WINTER NIGHTS when you wish you were living in Italy. It's a comfort soup through and through; every spoonful feels as though you are in Tuscany being embraced by the famous sunlight.

2 oz (56 g) prosciutto (4 to 5 slices) (see note)

1 Tbsp canola oil

1 onion, diced

6 cloves garlic, minced

3 stalks celery, leaves included, thinly sliced

2 medium carrots, scrubbed and cut in ½-inch slices

8 oz (225 g) cremini mushrooms, rinsed and thinly sliced

½ tsp table salt

¼ tsp freshly ground black pepper

1 (28 fl oz/796 mL) can no-salt-added San Marzano tomatoes

3 cups no-salt-added chicken broth

2 (19 fl oz/540 mL) cans no-salt-added cannellini or white kidney beans, rinsed and well drained

2 Mairlyn's Flavour Bombs (page 77) or ¼ cup store-bought pesto

3 cups baby kale or coarsely chopped kale, stalks removed

6 Tbsp finely grated Parmigiano-Reggiano

1. Chop the prosciutto into pieces the size of a white bean and set aside.

2. Heat a Dutch oven or a large saucepan over medium-high heat. Add the oil and prosciutto and sauté until the prosciutto starts to look cooked and the fat has melted off, 1 to 2 minutes.

3. Add the onion and continue sautéing until it starts to turn golden brown, 3 to 5 minutes. Add the garlic, celery, carrots, mushrooms, salt, and pepper and sauté for 3 to 5 minutes, until the vegetables begin to soften.

4. Add the tomatoes, broth, and beans. Stir well, scraping any browned bits off the bottom of the pot. Bring the soup to a boil, cover, and simmer for 20 to 25 minutes, until the carrots are soft.

5. Add the flavour bombs (or pesto) and kale and stir well. If using flavour bombs, allow them to melt. Remove the soup from the heat. Ladle into six individual bowls and sprinkle each serving with 1 Tbsp Parmigiano-Reggiano.

NOTE: Prosciutto is an Italian dry-cured ham that is usually thinly sliced and served uncooked or added to risottos or pasta dishes. I love the flavour it adds to this thick soup. Feel free to substitute either pancetta (an Italian style of bacon) or back bacon.

1 SERVING = 2 CUPS
PER SERVING: 371 CALORIES, 10.4 G TOTAL FAT, 2.1 G SATURATED FAT, 0 G TRANS FAT, 5 MG CHOLESTEROL, 562 MG SODIUM, 46.2 G CARBOHYDRATE, 11.9 G FIBRE, 7.1 G SUGARS, 0 G ADDED SUGARS, 23.2 G PROTEIN, 1328 MG POTASSIUM
CARBOHYDRATE CHOICE = 2 CHOICES

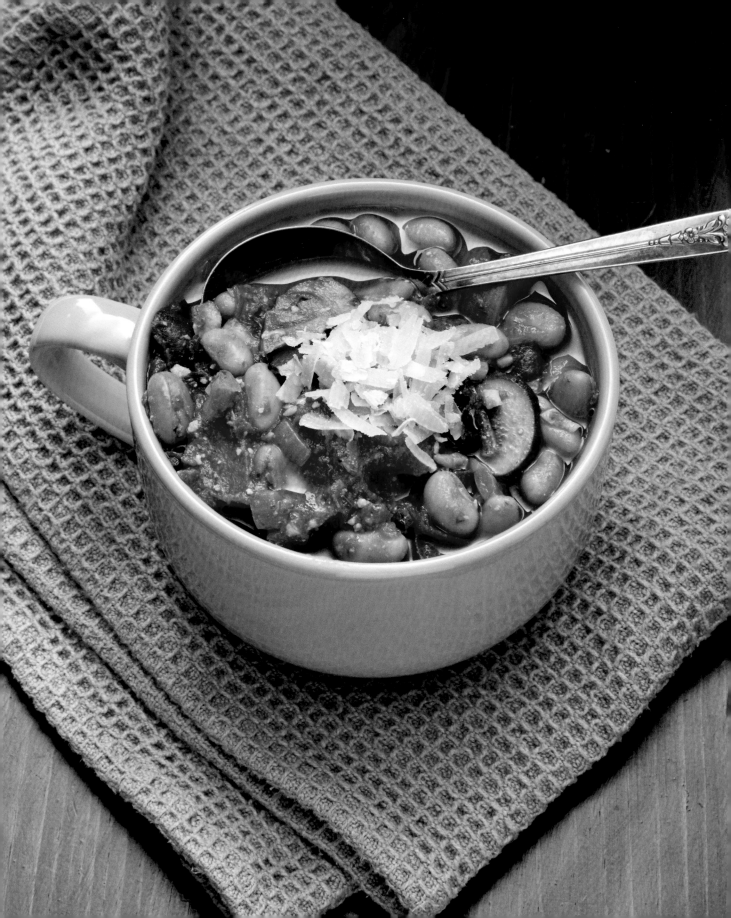

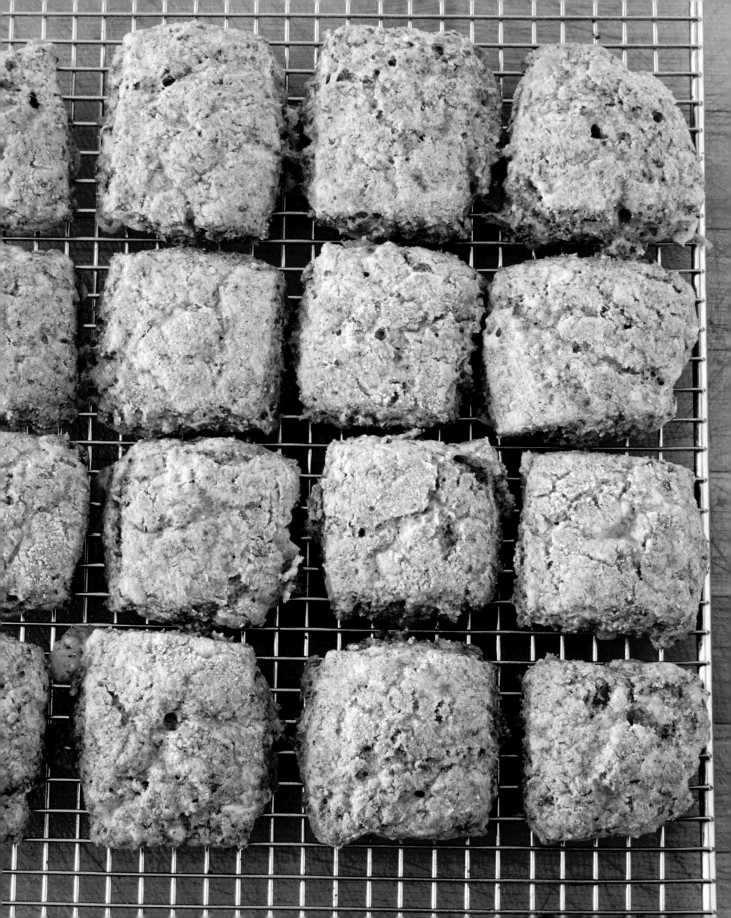

Cheddar Cheese Mini Dinner Biscuits *Makes 16 biscuits*

I HAVE THE GREATEST NEIGHBOURS. There are many summer nights when we end up having impromptu porch parties from around 8 p.m. until the wee hours. All my neighbours love taste-testing my recipes, but Evelyne has a special gift—she's a super taster. She can taste nuances and subtleties that most people can't. If Evelyne doesn't like something, I know it's *el crappo* and it's back to the drawing board for me. When I created this cheesy biscuit, I trotted some over to Evelyne's house. She took a couple of bites and then said without prompting, "There's a different flour in here . . ." Bingo, she was right, I had used whole grain barley to add some much-needed fibre. She's that good.

1½ cups + 2 Tbsp whole grain barley flour (divided)

½ cup flaxseed meal (see page 184)

⅛ to ¼ tsp freshly ground black pepper

1 Tbsp baking powder

¼ cup cold unsalted butter

1½ cups (5 oz/140 g) lightly packed grated 5-year-old white Cheddar cheese

½ cup skim milk

2 Tbsp canola oil

1 omega-3 egg

NOTE: Measure flour correctly: spoon the flour into a dry measuring cup (metal or plastic), then use a straight-edge kitchen tool, like a large metal spatula, to level it off (see page 188).

1. Make sure the rack in your oven is in the middle position. Preheat the oven to 375°F. Line a 9 × 13-inch rimless baking sheet with parchment paper. Set aside.

2. In a large bowl, whisk together 1½ cups barley flour, flaxseed meal, pepper and baking powder. Using a pastry cutter or two knives, cut in the butter until it's the size of small green peas. Using a fork, stir in the cheese until it's evenly distributed and coated in flour.

3. In a small bowl, whisk together the milk, oil, and egg. Pour the milk mixture into the dry ingredients and stir until it all comes together in a dough. The dough will be very sticky.

4. Sprinkle the remaining 2 Tbsp barley flour onto a clean counter and then tip out the dough. Gently knead the dough in the flour.

5. Pat the dough into a 5½ × 6½-inch rectangle and then cut it into 16 equal biscuits. Transfer to the prepared pan and bake for 14 to 16 minutes.

6. Remove the biscuits from the oven, let cool at least 5 minutes (or they will crumble), and serve.

1 SERVING = 1 BISCUIT
PER SERVING: 140 CALORIES, 9 G TOTAL FAT, 3.6 G SATURATED FAT, 0 G TRANS FAT, 20 MG CHOLESTEROL, 136 MG SODIUM, 10.4 G CARBOHYDRATE, 2.9 G FIBRE, 0.5 G SUGARS, 0 G ADDED SUGARS, 4.3 G PROTEIN, 97 MG POTASSIUM
CARBOHYDRATE CHOICE = ½ CHOICE

Cornbread VEG · *Serves 16*

I'VE NEVER BEEN A BIG FAN OF CORNBREAD. The ones I've tried were either too sweet or had no flavour at all, hence the slathering-on of the butter. People rave about their cornbread, so I kept trying to like it, but to no avail. Then I was doing some work with the Saskatchewan Mustard Development Commission (yes, there is such a wonderful marketing board), and they sent me a fabulous cookbook that had mustard in every recipe, including one for cornbread with ham and honey mustard. I set out to play using their recipe as a template and came up with something new. It totally changed my mind about cornbread—oh, the marvels of mustard. This goes well with the Spicy Slow-Cooker Vegetarian Chili (page 134) or the Skillet Enchiladas (page 150). You can see a picture of the Cornbread on page 150 as well.

1 cup medium-grind cornmeal (see note)

1 cup whole grain spelt flour

¼ cup flaxseed meal (see page 184)

1 Tbsp baking powder

1 Tbsp dry mustard

2 tsp yellow mustard seeds

⅛ tsp table salt

¼ tsp red pepper flakes

¼ tsp freshly ground black pepper

¾ cup skim milk

1 omega-3 egg

¼ cup canola oil

¼ cup liquid honey or pure amber maple syrup

2 Tbsp Dijon or yellow mustard

½ cup finely diced red onion

1 SERVING = 1 PIECE
PER SERVING: 128 CALORIES, 5.4 G TOTAL FAT, 0.6 G SATURATED FAT, 0 G TRANS FAT, 13 MG CHOLESTEROL, 119 MG SODIUM, 18.2 G CARBOHYDRATE, 2.3 G FIBRE, 5.5 G SUGARS, 4.4 G ADDED SUGARS, 3.1 G PROTEIN, 94 MG POTASSIUM
CARBOHYDRATE CHOICE = 1 CHOICE

1. Place a rack in the middle of the oven and preheat the oven to 425°F. Line an 8-inch square metal baking pan with wet parchment paper (see page 15).

2. In a large bowl, whisk together the cornmeal, spelt flour, flaxseed meal, baking powder, dry mustard, mustard seeds, salt, red pepper flakes, and pepper.

3. In a small bowl, whisk together the milk, egg, oil, honey or syrup, and mustard.

4. Add the red onion to the dry ingredients. Stir to coat. Pour in the wet ingredients and stir until well combined and there isn't any dry flour visible in the bowl. You can't overmix this, but having said that, don't go crazy and beat it.

5. Pour the batter into the prepared pan, making sure that the top is spread out evenly and that the batter reaches the edges of the pan. Bake for 20 to 25 minutes or until a toothpick inserted in the centre of the pan comes out clean.

6. Let the cornbread sit in the pan for 2 minutes, then cut it into 16 equal pieces. Serve right away.

NOTE: Is your cornmeal a whole grain? Check the label of your package of cornmeal for the answer. If the label says "degermed corn" anywhere, it isn't a whole grain, which will reduce the nutrient density and the fibre count. I prefer medium-grind cornmeal in baking for a rustic, slightly crunchy texture and its nutrient and fibre superiority. Cornmeal can be stored in the freezer for up to 2 years.

Irish Soda Bread VEG · *Serves 8*

THIS HEART-HEALTHY SPIN ON THE TRADITIONAL IRISH SODA BREAD is considered a quick bread in the world of home economics. It's bread-like but doesn't use yeast, so it's faster than prepping, kneading, proofing, rising, and baking a yeast bread. It's great with any of the dinner soups. See a picture on page 56.

2¼ cups + 2 Tbsp whole grain barley flour (divided)

2 Tbsp natural wheat germ

2 Tbsp flaxseed meal (see page 184)

1 tsp baking soda

1 omega-3 egg

¾ cup 1% buttermilk

2 Tbsp canola oil

1 Tbsp pure amber maple syrup

1. Make sure the rack in your oven is in the middle position. Preheat the oven to 350°F. Line a rimless baking sheet with parchment paper.

2. In a large bowl, whisk together the dry ingredients: 2¼ cups flour, wheat germ, flaxseed meal, and baking soda.

3. In a small bowl, whisk together the wet ingredients: egg, buttermilk, oil, and maple syrup.

4. Add the wet ingredients to the dry and stir using a large wooden spoon or a spatula. The dough is very sticky. Bring it together and form it into a ball.

5. Sprinkle a clean counter or wooden board with the remaining 2 Tbsp barley flour and tip the dough on top of the flour. Flatten and fold the ball in half and turn a quarter turn. Repeat three more times, flattening and folding and turning each time. Shape into a disc about 6 inches in diameter and ½ inch thick. Cut a shallow X in the centre of the disc.

6. Transfer the dough to the prepared baking sheet and bake for 32 to 36 minutes, until the top is cracked and the bottom is very brown. Remove the bread from the pan and place on a wire rack for 5 to 10 minutes, until cool enough to slice. Cut into eight equal wedges and serve.

1 SERVING = ⅛ OF THE BREAD
PER SERVING: 202 CALORIES, 5.3 G TOTAL FAT, 0.7 G SATURATED FAT, 0 G TRANS FAT, 71 MG CHOLESTEROL, 169 MG SODIUM, 31.6 G CARBOHYDRATE, 6.6 G FIBRE, 2.8 G SUGARS, 1.5 G ADDED SUGARS, 3.9 G PROTEIN, 221 MG POTASSIUM
CARBOHYDRATE CHOICE = 2 CHOICES

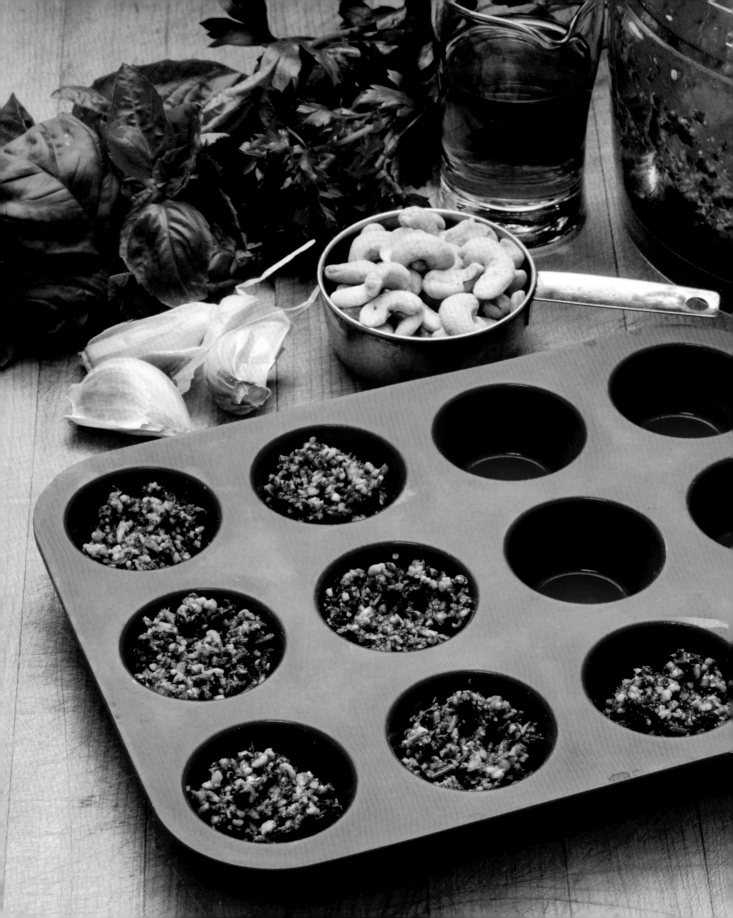

Mairlyn's Flavour Bombs VEG V LF GF · *Makes 1¼ cups*

FLAVOUR BOMBS ARE MY VERSION OF A CLASSIC PESTO. Pesto traditionally is made with basil, garlic, pine nuts, Parmigiano-Reggiano, and extra virgin olive oil. My flavour bombs have no cheese because my son is lactose-intolerant and I prefer the taste of cashews or walnuts in my pesto. I change up the oil depending on the nut I use. Pesto with cashews is all about a strong extra virgin olive oil to enhance the other ingredients. When I use walnuts, I use canola oil so the walnuts and basil shine through.

4 cups loosely packed fresh basil leaves or a combination of basil and parsley

6 cloves garlic

½ cup whole raw cashews or walnuts

½ cup extra virgin olive oil or canola oil

1. Rinse and pat dry the basil and parsley, if using, and line a large rimmed baking sheet with parchment paper or use silicone ice cube trays like I did in the photo.

2. Place the herbs in the bowl of a food processor fitted with the steel blade attachment. Add the garlic, nuts, and oil and process until well blended.

3. Scoop out 2 Tbsp portions and place them in balls on the baking sheet or in the silicone ice cube trays.

4. Freeze the flavour bombs in a flat layer. Once they're frozen, transfer them to a resealable freezer bag. They'll keep for up to 6 months.

1 SERVING = 2 TBSP
PER SERVING: 138 CALORIES, 13.9 G TOTAL FAT, 2 G SATURATED FAT, 0 G TRANS FAT, 0 MG CHOLESTEROL, 11 MG SODIUM, 3 G CARBOHYDRATE, 0.5 G FIBRE, 0.4 G SUGARS, 0 G ADDED SUGARS, 1.7 G PROTEIN, 120 MG POTASSIUM
CARBOHYDRATE CHOICE = < 1 CHOICE

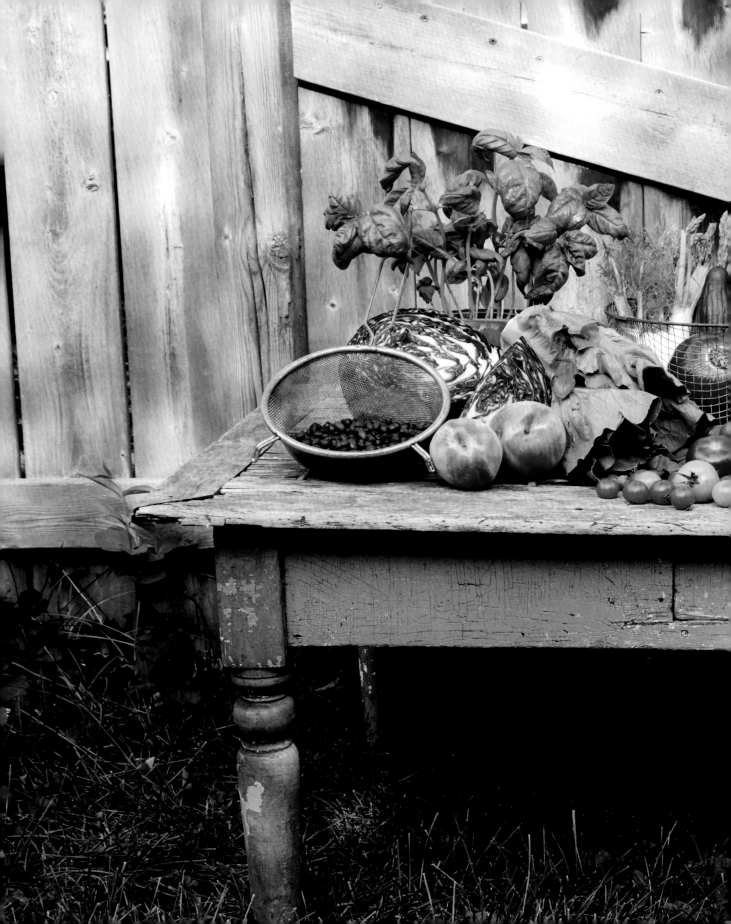

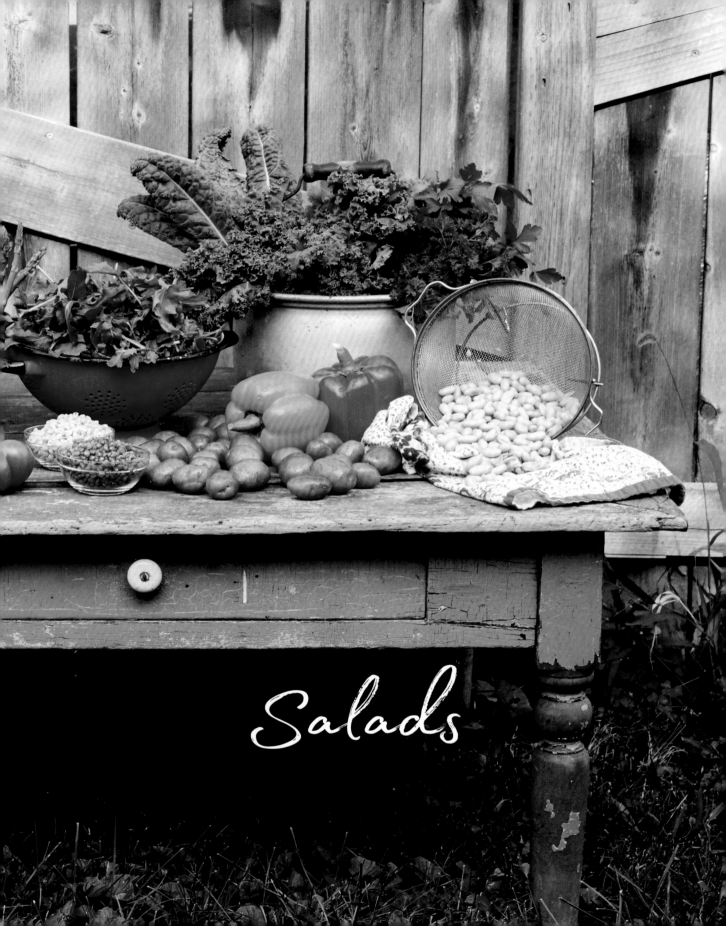

Salads

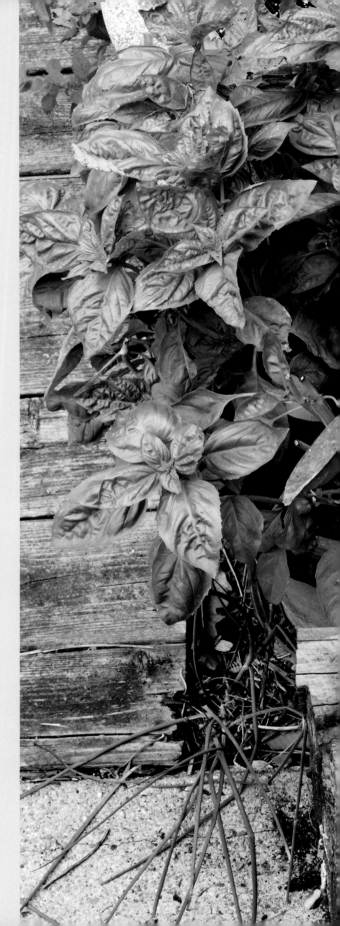

If your definition of a salad is a head of iceberg lettuce, a couple of chopped tomatoes, and some slices of cucumber drowned in white creamy salad dressing, this chapter might just blow your mind. There is nary an iceberg lettuce leaf to be seen, and only a couple of recipes use lettuce at all.

My salads are an eclectic assortment of fresh, seasonal ingredients. They're meant to encourage you and your family to add more fibre to your everyday meals through a variety of vegetables, fruits, grains, pulses, and leafy greens like kale and arugula. Salads are Mother Nature at her best.

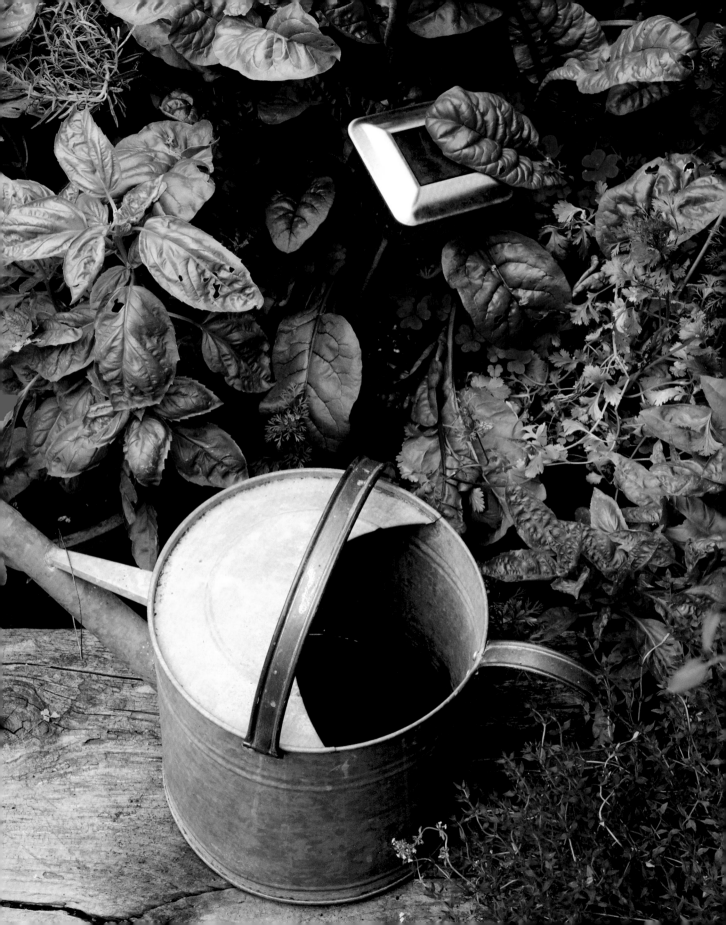

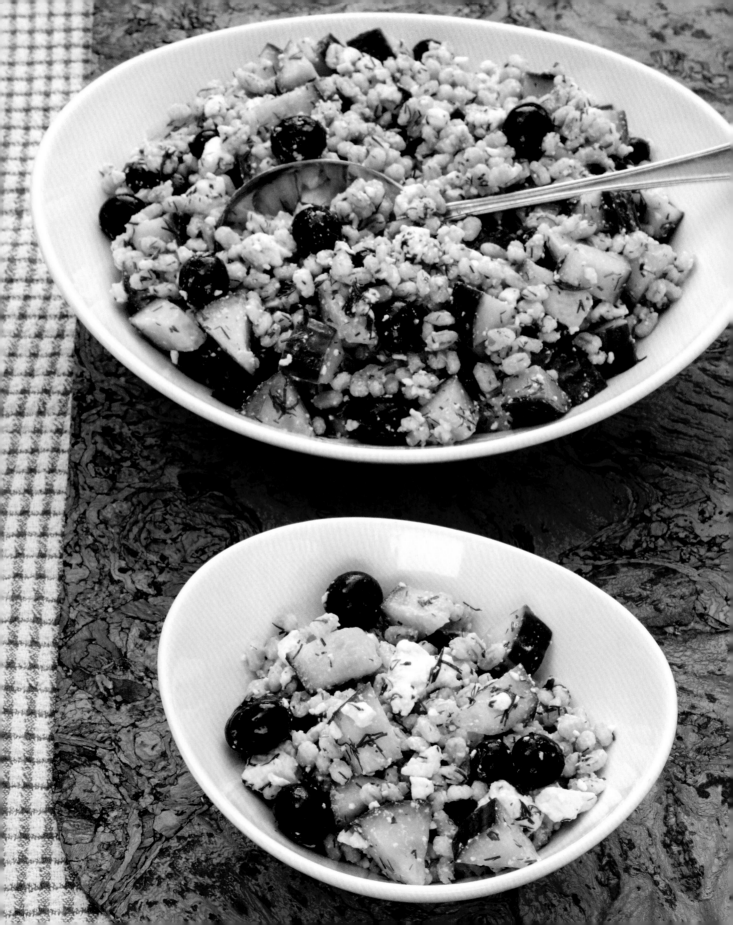

Blueberry Salad with Barley & Dill VEG · *Serves 8 as a side*

I'M A BLUEBERRY GIRL. I love those purple-blue orbs for their fabulous taste of summer and their high content of vitamins, minerals, antioxidants, and fibre. I don't love them quite as much when they stain my white T-shirts, but you need to take the bad with the good. When looking for the freshest blueberries, make sure they have a silver sheen on them. It's called bloom and it's an indication that they were just picked. No bloom? No buy.

SALAD DRESSING

2 Tbsp red wine vinegar

2 Tbsp extra virgin olive oil or canola oil

SALAD

1½ cups diced English cucumber (about ½ cucumber)

1½ to 1¾ cups cooked pot barley (see page 13)

½ cup chopped fresh dill

1 cup fresh local or wild blueberries, rinsed well and patted dry

½ cup (3 oz/85 g) crumbled feta cheese

1. Make the salad dressing. In a large bowl, whisk together the vinegar and oil.

2. Add the cucumbers, cooked barley, dill, blueberries, and feta. Toss well and serve right away.

NOTE: I cook a large pot of barley most weeks and then use the leftovers as a side dish or as an ingredient in salads.

1 SERVING = ½ CUP
PER SERVING: 117 CALORIES, 5.8 G TOTAL FAT, 2 G SATURATED FAT, 0 G TRANS FAT, 9 MG CHOLESTEROL, 93 MG SODIUM, 14.3 G CARBOHYDRATE, 2 G FIBRE, 2.8 G SUGARS, 0 G ADDED SUGARS, 2.5 G PROTEIN, 96 MG POTASSIUM
CARBOHYDRATE CHOICE = 1 CHOICE

Cold Soba Noodles with Cucumber & Ginger Sesame Dressing

VEG V LF · *Serves 6 as a side*

THE FIRST TIME I TRIED COLD SOBA NOODLES WAS AT A LITTLE JAPANESE RESTAURANT on Baldwin Street in Toronto. They came beautifully presented in a bowl on a bamboo mat. After my first bite, I knew I had to figure out how to make them. I decided to Mairlyn-ize the whole shebang, mainly because I couldn't find any bamboo mats. I serve the cold noodles in Asian-style bowls with cucumbers, green onions, and cilantro on top, drizzled with the dressing. The soba noodles need at least an hour to chill, so cook them in the morning or the night before and let them cool in the fridge until you need them for dinner.

SALAD DRESSING

3 Tbsp natural rice vinegar

3 Tbsp lower-sodium or lite tamari

2 Tbsp mirin

1 Tbsp grated fresh ginger

1 Tbsp sesame oil

⅛ tsp red pepper flakes

SALAD

2 bundles (about 6½ oz/185 g) buckwheat soba noodles (see note on page 66)

½ large English cucumber

3 green onions, whites included, thinly sliced

½ cup chopped fresh cilantro leaves

NOTE: This cold summer salad is perfect to serve with an Asian-flavoured chicken, pork, or salmon dish.

1. Make the salad dressing. In a 1-cup mason jar with a screw-top lid, whisk together the rice vinegar, tamari, mirin, ginger, oil, and red pepper flakes. Set aside or store in the fridge until you are making the salad.

2. Cook the soba noodles according to the package instructions. Drain into a colander, rinse gently under cold water, and continue to drain for at least 5 minutes. When fully drained, transfer the noodles to a container that has a tight-fitting lid, then drizzle 6 Tbsp dressing (for the math geeks, that's ¼ cup + 2 Tbsp) over the noodles and toss gently. Cover with the lid and chill in the fridge for at least 1 hour or overnight.

3. To prepare the cucumber, rinse it well, pat dry, and, leaving the peel on, cut it in half lengthwise. Slice into thin half moons and either use right away or store, covered, in the fridge overnight.

4. At serving time, you'll need six Asian-style or small bowls. Toss the noodles once more, then divide them equally among the bowls. It's about ¾ cup per serving. Equally divide the cucumbers, green onions, and cilantro and place on top of each pile of noodles. Drizzle the remaining salad dressing equally over top and serve.

1 SERVING = ⅙ OF THE RECIPE
PER SERVING: 149 CALORIES, 2.6 G TOTAL FAT, 0.4 G SATURATED FAT, 0 G TRANS FAT, 0 MG CHOLESTEROL, 520 MG SODIUM, 28.1 G CARBOHYDRATE, 1 G FIBRE, 4.2 G SUGARS, 0.5 G ADDED SUGARS, 5.6 G PROTEIN, 166 MG POTASSIUM
CARBOHYDRATE CHOICE = 2 CHOICES

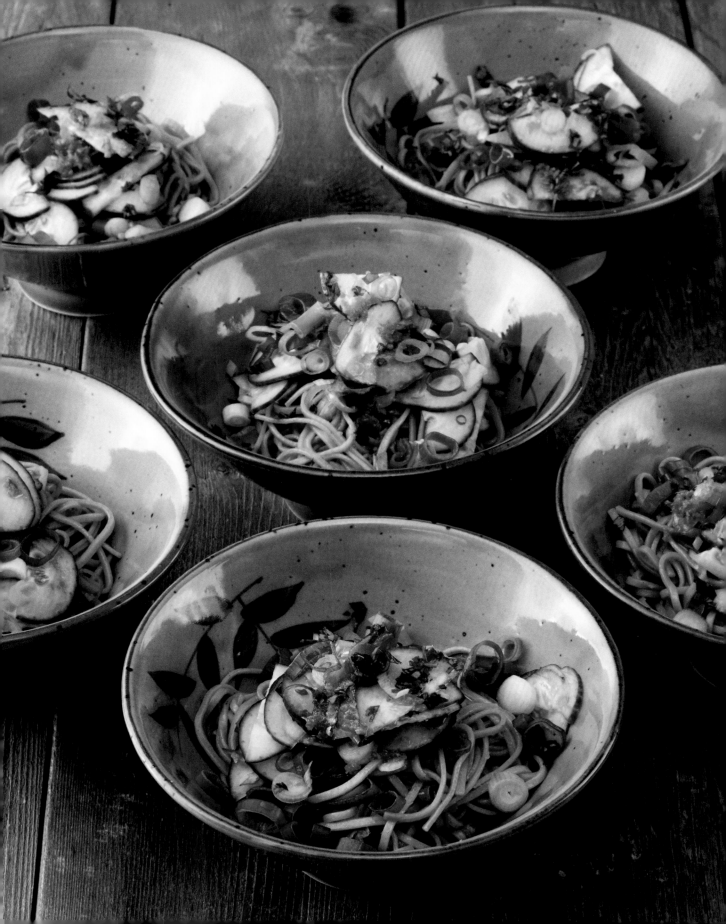

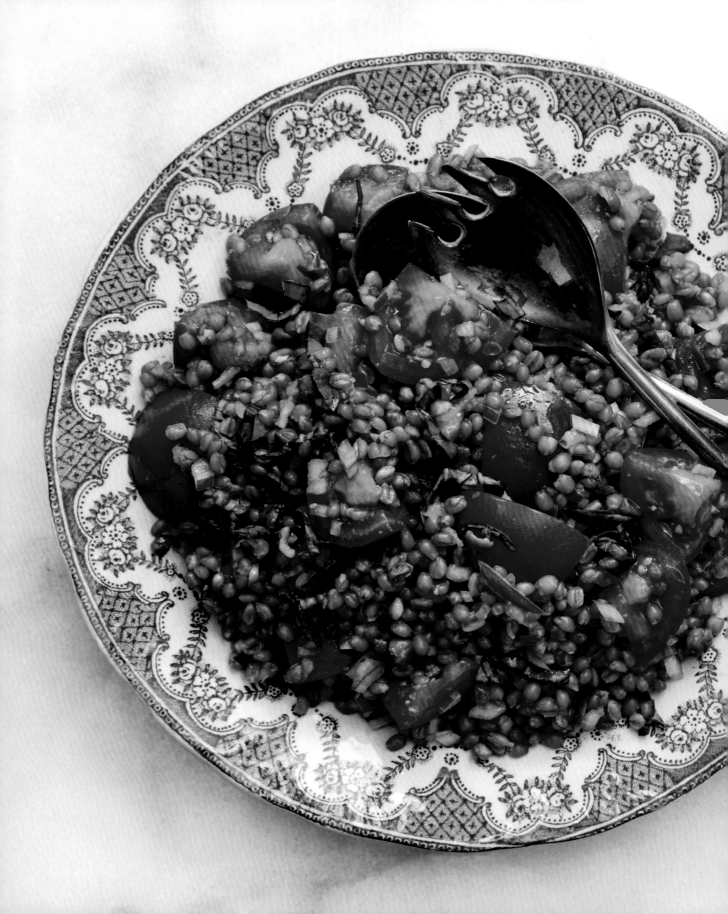

Italian Bread Salad without the Bread VEG V LF · *Serves 6 as a side*

EVERY ITALIAN HOME COOK KNOWS HOW TO CREATE A NEW RECIPE WITH LEFTOVERS.
Panzanella, an Italian bread salad, is made with stale bread kicking around the kitchen plus tomatoes, basil, and oil. In my case, I had leftover wheat berries that I didn't want to waste. And after all, wheat berries are the beginnings of bread . . . see where I'm going with this? This salad tastes great served with either grilled steak or chicken.

SALAD DRESSING

2 Tbsp extra virgin olive oil

2 Tbsp red wine vinegar

1 clove garlic, crushed

SALAD

½ cup diced red onion

5 ripe cocktail or Kumato tomatoes, cut in eighths (see note)

½ cup fresh basil leaves, torn into small pieces

2 Tbsp capers, drained, rinsed, and coarsely chopped

2 cups cooked wheat berries (see page 13)

1. Make the salad dressing. In a large bowl, whisk together the oil, vinegar, and garlic. Crushing releases the most flavour, so a little clove will go a long way in this salad.

2. Add the onion, tomatoes, basil, and capers and toss gently but well. You don't want the tomatoes to go all mushy. Add the wheat berries, toss gently, and serve.

NOTE: Kumato tomatoes are a naturally brown-skinned cocktail tomato that are sweet and firm and fabulous.

1 SERVING = ¾ CUP
PER SERVING: 116 CALORIES, 4.4 G TOTAL FAT, 0.6 G SATURATED FAT, 0 G TRANS FAT,
0 MG CHOLESTEROL, 62 MG SODIUM, 16.7 G CARBOHYDRATE, 3.3 G FIBRE, 1.4 G SUGARS,
0 G ADDED SUGARS, 4 G PROTEIN, 181 MG POTASSIUM
CARBOHYDRATE CHOICE = 1 CHOICE

Romaine with Buttermilk Ranch Dressing & Spicy Roasted Chickpeas VEG GF • *Serves 4 as a side*

I'VE EATEN SPICY CHICKPEAS AS A SNACK, but it wasn't until I had them in a salad that my chickpea snacking habit changed. Chef Massimo Capra serves a salad with crispy chickpeas at his restaurant Boccone Trattoria, at Toronto Pearson International Airport, and when I first tasted it, I knew I had to start adding them to my salads. They are a gluten-free alternative to croutons and a good source of protein, and then there's the fibre—don't forget the fibre. It's a triple win if you are living with celiac disease or are gluten-sensitive, and a double win for the rest of us mortals. No matter how you look at it, it's a win.

ROASTED CHICKPEAS

1 (19 fl oz/540 mL) can no-salt-added chickpeas, rinsed and well drained

2 Tbsp canola oil

½ to 1 tsp chipotle chili powder

1 large head romaine lettuce

SALAD DRESSING

3 Tbsp low-fat mayo (see sidebar)

3 Tbsp 0% plain Greek yogurt

¼ cup + 2 Tbsp 1% buttermilk

2 Tbsp finely chopped fresh dill

1 Tbsp finely chopped fresh parsley, leaves and stems

1 Tbsp finely chopped fresh chives

1 small clove garlic, crushed

¼ tsp freshly ground black pepper

ONE SERVING = ¼ OF THE SALAD
PER SERVING: 257 CALORIES, 12.7 G TOTAL
FAT, 1.4 G SATURATED FAT, 0 G TRANS FAT,
4 MG CHOLESTEROL, 254 MG SODIUM,
28 G CARBOHYDRATE, 7.3 G FIBRE,
4.3 G SUGARS, 0.4 G ADDED SUGARS,
9.6 G PROTEIN, 544 MG POTASSIUM
CARBOHYDRATE CHOICE = 1½ CHOICES

1. The chickpeas need to be dry to roast properly, so after you've rinsed and drained them, lay them out on a clean dish towel or paper towels and pat dry. If you aren't pressed for time, let them air-dry for at least 30 minutes.

2. When they are dry, preheat the oven to 400°F. Line a large rimmed baking sheet with parchment paper.

3. Place the chickpeas in a medium bowl, add the canola oil and toss to coat. Depending on how spicy you want them to be, sprinkle on ½ to 1 tsp of chili powder and mix well. Transfer the chickpeas to the prepared baking sheet and spread them out well. They need good air circulation to turn into crispy, yummy croutons. If they are crowded in the pan, they won't crisp up.

4. Roast for 30 to 45 minutes, turning them in the pan at the 30-minute mark. They need to be really browned to be crispy. If they aren't brown, then pop them back in the oven.

5. Meanwhile, rinse and spin-dry the lettuce in a salad spinner or pat dry with clean paper towels or a tea towel. Tear the lettuce into bite-sized pieces, and set aside in the fridge.

6. Make the salad dressing. In a 2-cup mason jar or a medium bowl, shake or whisk together the mayo, yogurt, buttermilk, dill, parsley, chives, garlic, and pepper. Store in the fridge until serving time.

7. When the chickpeas are roasted, remove them from the oven and then, very carefully, pick up the parchment paper by all four corners and transfer the whole thing, parchment paper and all, onto a wire cooling rack. This is an important step in the crunchy process, as the chickpeas tend to get slightly soggy when cooling in the pan.

8. When the chickpeas are cool, after about 15 minutes, get the romaine and the salad dressing out of the fridge and toss together. Add the chickpeas, toss well, and divide equally among four large salad bowls. Garnish with extra freshly ground pepper if desired.

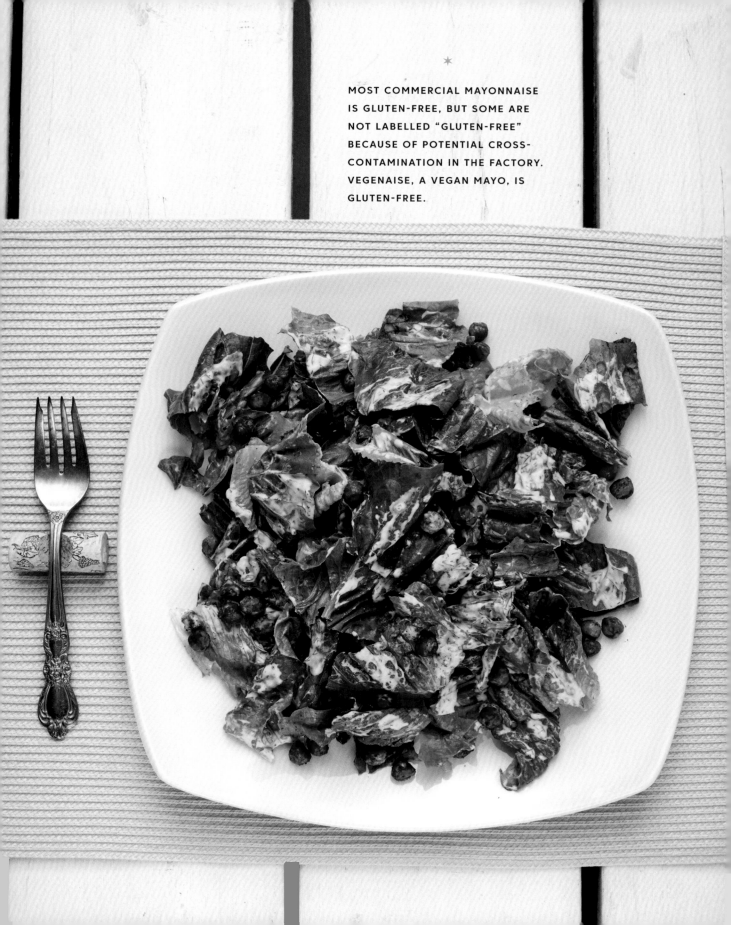

MOST COMMERCIAL MAYONNAISE
IS GLUTEN-FREE, BUT SOME ARE
NOT LABELLED "GLUTEN-FREE"
BECAUSE OF POTENTIAL CROSS-
CONTAMINATION IN THE FACTORY.
VEGENAISE, A VEGAN MAYO, IS
GLUTEN-FREE.

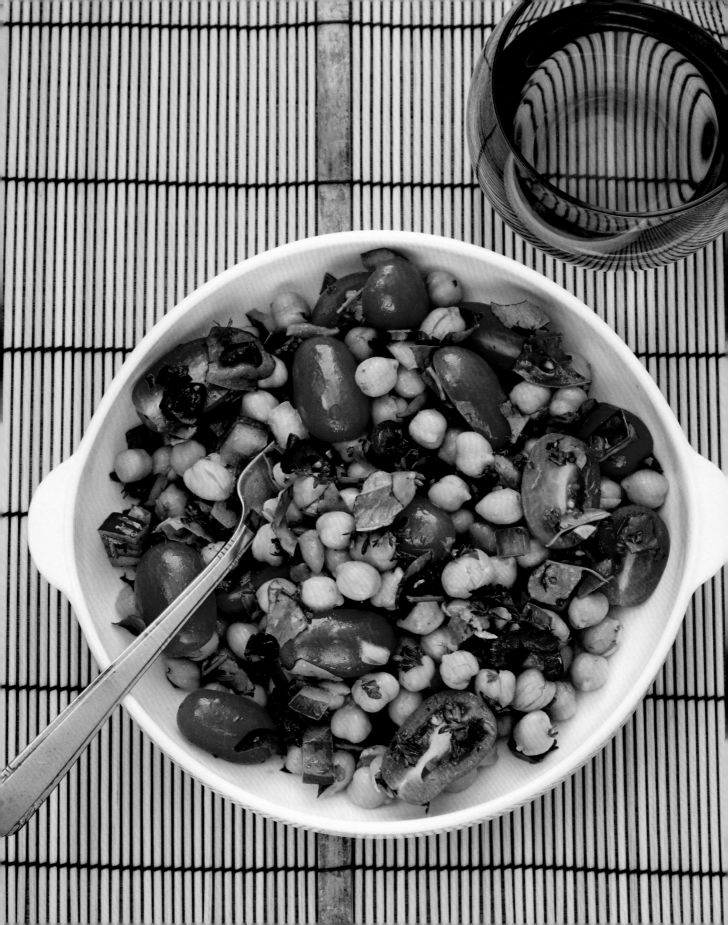

Smith Summer Favourite Chickpea Salad VEG V LF GF · *Serves 4 as a side*

THE TWO THINGS YOU'LL ALWAYS FIND IN MY FRIDGE IN THE SUMMER are a bottle of sparkling white wine and a can of chickpeas. Sparkling white wine, because you never know when you want to celebrate something, but chickpeas? What's with that? As a professional home economist, I'm always trying to make your life easier in the kitchen. Storing a can of unopened chickpeas in the fridge during the summer months means that you can toss together a vegetarian salad quickly because the chickpeas are already cold. It's a salad game changer.

SALAD DRESSING

1 clove garlic, diced

1 to 2 Tbsp La Bomba antipasto spread (see page 11)

2 Tbsp extra virgin olive oil

2 Tbsp red wine vinegar

SALAD

1 (19 fl oz/540 mL) can no-salt-added chickpeas, rinsed and well drained

2 cups grape tomatoes, halved

1 cup fresh basil leaves, rinsed, patted dry, and torn into small pieces

¼ cup finely chopped fresh parsley leaves

¼ cup diced red onion

18 Kalamata olives, pitted and coarsely chopped

1. Make the salad dressing. In a large bowl, whisk together the garlic, La Bomba, oil, and vinegar.

2. Add the chickpeas, tomatoes, basil, parsley, red onion, and olives. Toss well. Serve or store in the fridge for up to 2 days. This tastes amazing served with a whole grain baguette.

NOTE: To make this a vegetarian or vegan entrée, you can increase the serving size to 2½ cups per person. Trust me, you'll be full of beans.

1 SERVING = 1¼ CUPS
PER SERVING: 254 CALORIES, 14.2 G TOTAL FAT, 1.9 G SATURATED FAT, 0 G TRANS FAT, 0 MG CHOLESTEROL, 472 MG SODIUM, 25.8 G CARBOHYDRATE, 5.2 G FIBRE, 3.1 G SUGARS, 0 G ADDED SUGARS, 6.8 G PROTEIN, 295 MG POTASSIUM
CARBOHYDRATE CHOICE = 1½ CHOICES

White Bean Summer Salad VEG GF · *Serves 5 as a side*

I GROW POTS OF MINT, PARSLEY, BASIL, OREGANO, THYME, AND ROSEMARY outside my back door. It makes me happy whenever I step outside and can add some fresh flavours and antioxidants to my food. As mentioned for chickpeas in the recipe introduction on page 91, I'd encourage you to store an unopened can of white kidney beans in your fridge throughout the hot summer months. Want a quick dinner? Just open, rinse, drain, and throw into a big green salad, and dinner is ready.

SALAD DRESSING

3 Tbsp canola oil or extra virgin olive oil

3 Tbsp apple cider vinegar

2 cloves garlic, minced

1 Tbsp grainy Dijon mustard

2 tsp pure amber maple syrup

⅛ tsp table salt

SALAD

1 (19 fl oz/540 mL) can no-salt-added white kidney beans, rinsed and well drained

1 stalk celery, diced

1 red pepper, diced

1 cup roughly chopped fresh parsley, leaves and stems (see note)

¼ cup thinly sliced fresh mint leaves

½ cup diced red onion

½ cup (3 oz/85 g) crumbled feta cheese

NOTE: If the herbs are too wet, the salad loses some of its flavour. Rinse the herbs under cold running water, then spin them in a salad spinner or pat them dry with a clean tea towel before chopping.

1. Make the salad dressing. In a large bowl, whisk together the oil, vinegar, garlic, mustard, maple syrup, and salt.

2. Add the drained white beans, celery, red pepper, parsley, mint, red onion, and feta. Toss well. Serve right away or store in the fridge for up to 3 days. This is a great dish to pack for a picnic (see picture on the opposite page).

1 SERVING = 1 CUP
PER SERVING: 246 CALORIES, 12.6 G TOTAL FAT, 3.7 G SATURATED FAT, 0 G TRANS FAT, 15 MG CHOLESTEROL, 265 MG SODIUM, 23.4 G CARBOHYDRATE, 6.1 G FIBRE, 3.7 G SUGARS, 0.8 G ADDED SUGARS, 10.5 G PROTEIN, 426 MG POTASSIUM
CARBOHYDRATE CHOICE = 1 CHOICE

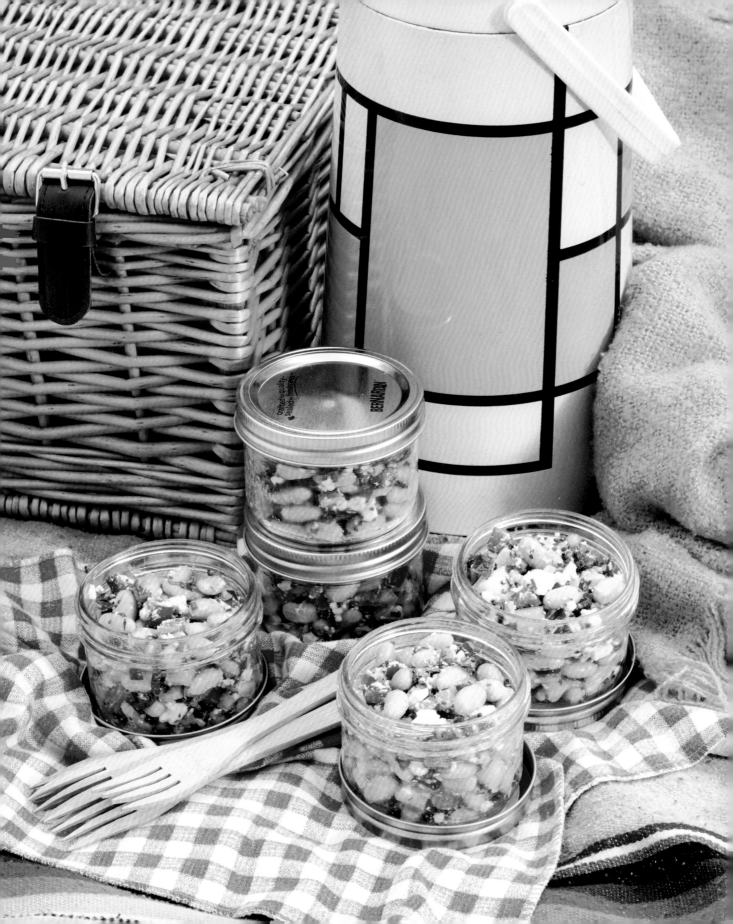

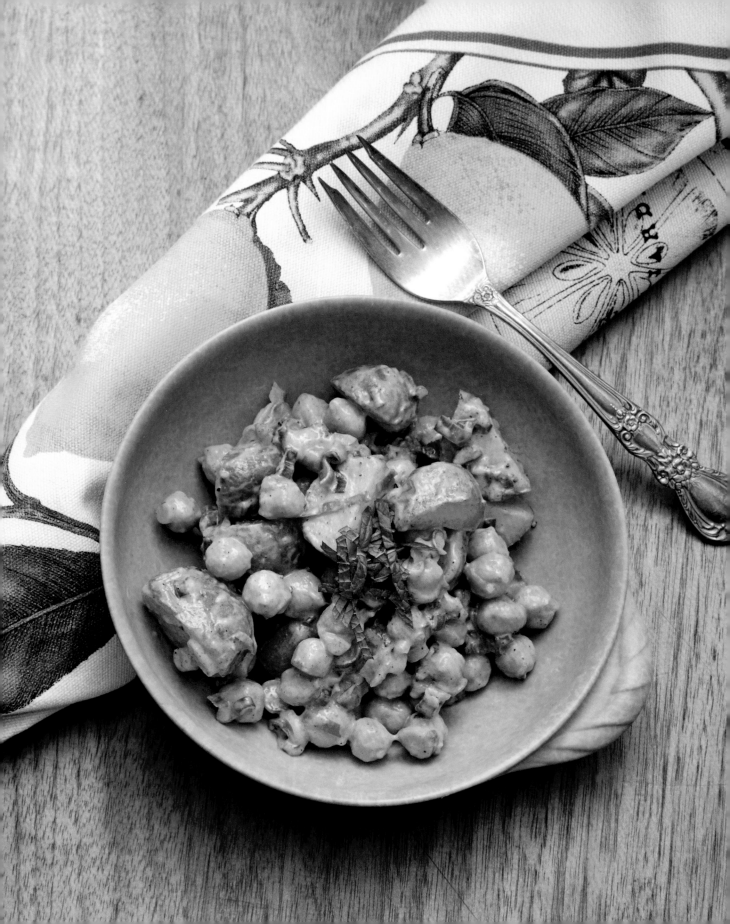

Curried Chickpea & Potato Salad VEG · *Serves 12 as a side*

FOR THE RECORD, I DON'T HAVE ANYTHING AGAINST TRADITIONAL POTATO SALAD. My mom made a fabulous one with gobs of mayo, hard-cooked eggs, onions, and potatoes. It's just that I love trying new spins and flavour combinations more than I love gobs of mayo. Which explains why both salads that use potatoes in this cookbook are out there in left field. Don't expect your mama's potato salad when you are making a Mairlyn potato salad!

SALAD

1½ lb (680 g) small red-skinned new potatoes, rinsed well, skin on

1 bunch green onions, whites included, thinly sliced

1 (19 fl oz/540 mL) can no-salt-added chickpeas, rinsed and well drained

½ cup thinly sliced fresh mint leaves

SALAD DRESSING

¼ cup low-fat mayo

¼ cup 2% plain yogurt

2 tsp medium curry powder

¼ tsp ground turmeric

½ tsp freshly ground black pepper

½ tsp table salt

2 Tbsp spicy mango chutney

1 SERVING = ½ CUP
PER SERVING: 101 CALORIES, 2.1 G TOTAL FAT, 0.3 G SATURATED FAT, 0 G TRANS FAT, 1 MG CHOLESTEROL, 139 MG SODIUM, 17.8 G CARBOHYDRATE, 2.8 G FIBRE, 3.9 G SUGARS, 1.8 G ADDED SUGARS, 3.5 G PROTEIN, 336 MG POTASSIUM
CARBOHYDRATE CHOICE = 1 CHOICE

1. Place a steamer basket inside a medium-sized saucepan and add enough water so that the water is barely touching the bottom of the steamer. Place the potatoes inside the basket. Heat on medium-high and bring the water to a boil. Once boiling, cover the pot and cook until the potatoes are fork-tender. Depending on the size, this can take 10 to 15 minutes. Check the water level to make sure they don't boil dry. When the potatoes are just tender, remove the pot from the heat, remove the lid, and let cool.

2. While the potatoes are cooking, make the salad dressing. In a large bowl, whisk together the mayo, yogurt, curry powder, turmeric, pepper, and salt. Stir in the mango chutney.

3. Add the green onions and chickpeas to the dressing and toss well.

4. When the potatoes are cool enough to handle, remove them from the steamer basket. Depending on the size of these wee beauties, you can cut them into halves or into quarters. They should be about the size of four chickpeas lumped together. The big tip is that you don't want the potatoes to overpower the chickpeas in size or flavour. Add the potatoes and mint to the bowl of chickpeas and toss well. Refrigerate for at least 8 hours or overnight to create resistant starch in the salad (see note). Serve cold.

NOTE: Starchy foods such as potatoes have been getting a bad rap for years, but luckily for potato lovers, a newly appreciated component called resistant starch is making the news, and cooked cold potatoes are a source of this type of starch. For more information, see page 3.

Potato & Asparagus Salad with Basil & Arugula Pesto

VEG V LF GF · *Serves 8 as a side*

I KNOW THERE ARE POTATOES IN THIS SALAD, but trust me, this is *not* a potato salad. This is a salad with potatoes for all those people who think outside the potato salad box, seeing possibilities with potatoes and other vegetables and absolutely no mayo. This salad needs to cool before being eaten, so if you want it for dinner tonight, get those potatoes cooking right now.

SALAD

1½ lb (680 g) mini red-skinned potatoes, rinsed, skin on

1 lb (450 g) fresh local asparagus, trimmed of coarse woody stalks

½ cup diced red onion

24 Kalamata olives, pitted and coarsely chopped

PESTO

3 Tbsp extra virgin olive oil or canola oil

4 cloves garlic

1 cup packed baby arugula, rinsed and patted dry

1 cup packed fresh basil, leaves and stems, rinsed and patted dry

½ tsp table salt

¼ tsp freshly ground black pepper

1 SERVING = 1 CUP
PER SERVING: 136 CALORIES, 7.9 G TOTAL FAT, 0.7 G SATURATED FAT, 0 G TRANS FAT, 0 MG CHOLESTEROL, 376 MG SODIUM, 15.5 G CARBOHYDRATE, 2.8 G FIBRE, 3.5 G SUGARS, 0 G ADDED SUGARS, 3.1 G PROTEIN, 519 MG POTASSIUM
CARBOHYDRATE CHOICE = 1 CHOICE

1. Place a steamer basket inside a medium-sized saucepan and add enough water so that the water is barely touching the bottom of the steamer. Place the potatoes inside the basket. Heat on medium-high and bring the water to a boil. Once boiling, cover the pot and cook until the potatoes are fork-tender. Depending on the size, this can take 10 to 15 minutes. Check the water level to make sure they don't boil dry. When the potatoes are just tender, remove the pot from the heat, remove the lid, and tip into a colander to cool.

2. Once the potatoes are cooked, rinse the asparagus and, using the same saucepan and steamer, place the asparagus into the steamer basket and back into the saucepan. Add enough water so that the water is barely touching the bottom of the steamer. Heat on medium-high and bring the water to a boil. Once boiling, cover the pot and steam for 3 to 5 minutes, until the asparagus is bright green and slightly tender. Drain the asparagus and immediately run it under very cold water. When the asparagus is no longer too hot to handle, 2 to 3 minutes, place it on a clean tea towel and gently pat dry.

3. Place the cooked potatoes and asparagus in covered containers and refrigerate until cold. It's best to do this overnight.

4. Make the pesto. In the bowl of a food processor fitted with the steel blade attachment, pulse the oil, garlic, arugula, basil, salt, and pepper until well combined. Pour into a small container and store in the fridge.

5. To serve, cut the asparagus into 1-inch pieces, leaving the tops intact. Cut the cold potatoes into quarters. In a large bowl, toss together the asparagus, potatoes, red onion, and olives. Add the pesto and toss well to coat. Serve right away or cover and refrigerate for up to 24 hours.

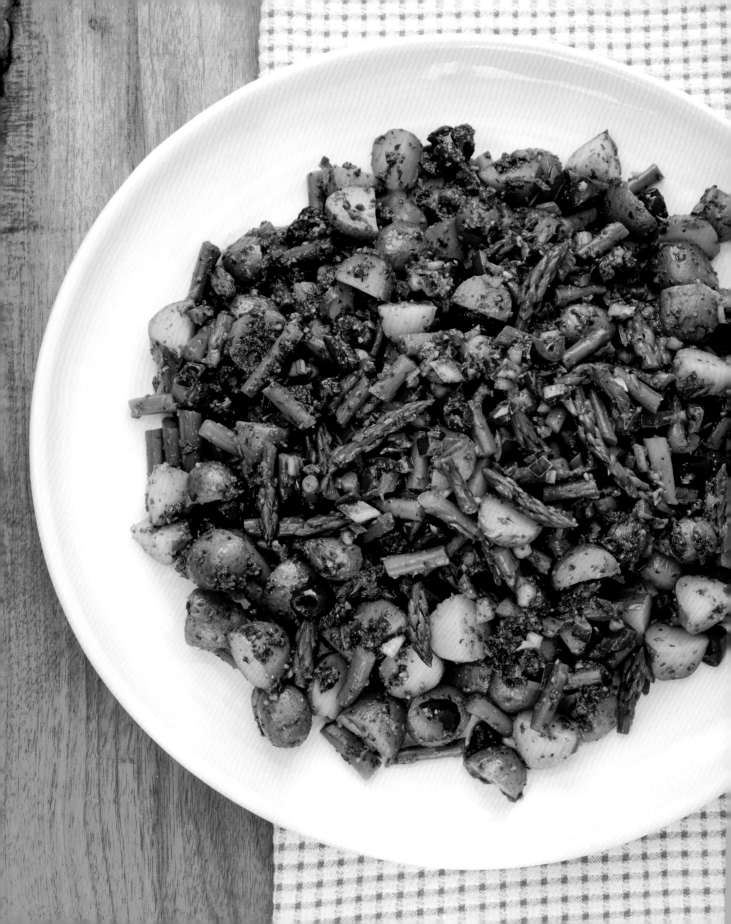

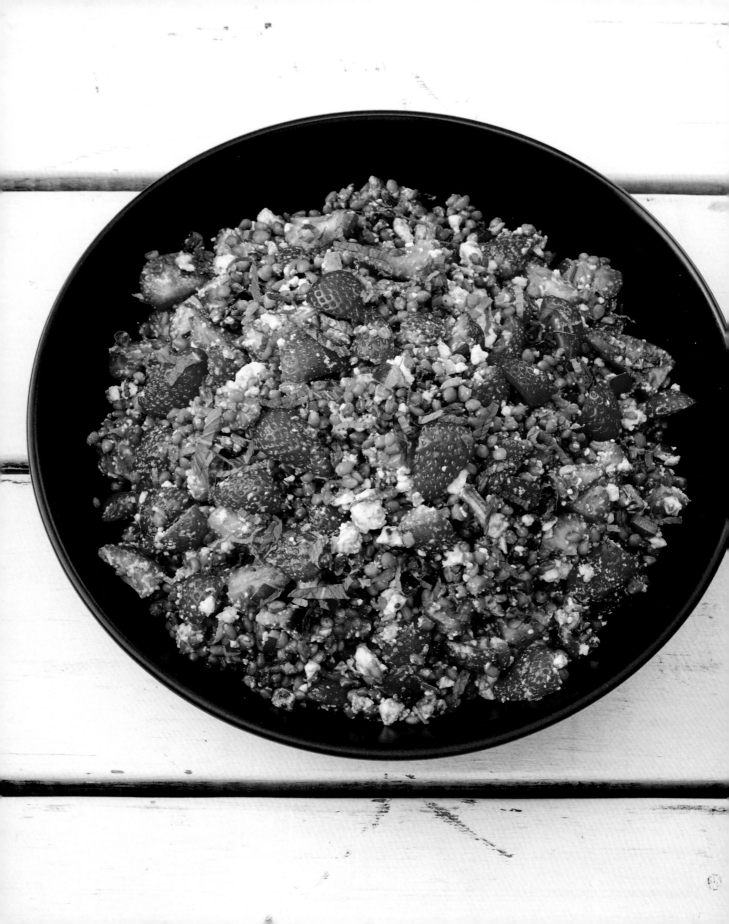

Lentil & Wheat Berry Salad with Strawberries & Mint

VEG · *Serves 16 as a side*

I GET MY INSPIRATION FOR NEW RECIPES AFTER EATING IN A RESTAURANT, watching a cooking show, surfing YouTube or Pinterest, or from real moments in time. Case in point: this recipe was inspired when my assistant, Katie, was over helping me prep for one of my *Cityline* segments and both of us were hungry, bordering on *hangry*. I had some leftover cooked lentils in my fridge, so I threw together a quick dinner salad with some other ingredients I had kicking around, followed up with a splash of oil and vinegar, and voilà, a recipe was born.

1¾ cups chilled cooked wheat berries (see page 13)

SALAD DRESSING
¼ cup balsamic vinegar

3 Tbsp extra virgin olive oil

2 tsp Dijon mustard

SALAD
1 (19 fl oz/540 mL) can lentils, rinsed and well drained

1 cup thinly sliced fresh mint leaves

1 cup diced red onion

1 cup (6 oz/170 g) crumbled feta cheese

3 cups strawberries, rinsed, patted dry, tops removed, and quartered

✳

PROFESSIONAL HOME ECONOMIST TIP: I usually cook a pot of whole grains or quinoa, which is technically a seed, to have on hand for dinners. If you don't have cooked wheat berries kicking around in your fridge, check out page 13 for the directions.

1. Make sure your cooked wheat berries are cold—if needed, chill at least 4 hours or overnight.

2. When the wheat berries have chilled, start making the salad dressing. In a large bowl, whisk together the vinegar, oil, and Dijon.

3. Add the wheat berries, lentils, mint, and red onion, and toss well. Fold in the feta. Just before serving, add the strawberries, gently combine, and enjoy.

1 SERVING = ½ CUP
PER SERVING: 129 CALORIES, 5.2 G TOTAL FAT, 1.7 G SATURATED FAT, 0 G TRANS FAT, 9 MG CHOLESTEROL, 164 MG SODIUM, 16 G CARBOHYDRATE, 3.3 G FIBRE, 2.8 G SUGARS, 0 G ADDED SUGARS, 4.2 G PROTEIN, 197 MG POTASSIUM
CARBOHYDRATE CHOICE = 1 CHOICE

Peaches & Arugula Salad VEG GF · *Serves 2 as a light main or 4 as a side*

ONLY WHEN LOCAL PEACHES ARE AT THEIR HEIGHT OF JUICY, luscious perfection do I give you permission to make this summer salad. Plate this simply by layering the ingredients as they appear in the recipe. Finish with a drizzle of oil and vinegar, and it's ready. To serve it as a light main, try adding some grilled chicken or pork.

4 cups baby arugula or baby arugula/spinach mix, rinsed and spun dry

3 ripe peaches, peeled and sliced

½ cup (3 oz/85 g) crumbled feta cheese

¼ cup diced red onion

2 Tbsp whole raw almonds, coarsely chopped

¼ cup fresh whole mint leaves, rinsed and patted dry

2 to 4 Tbsp extra virgin olive oil or canola oil (see note)

2 to 4 Tbsp apple cider vinegar

1. Get out two large dinner plates (or four salad plates if serving this as an appetizer or side). Divide the arugula evenly onto each plate.

2. Divide the sliced peaches evenly between the plates. Sprinkle with the feta, red onion, and almonds. Tear the mint leaves into small pieces and top the salads.

3. Drizzle each plate with 1 Tbsp oil and then drizzle each with 1 Tbsp vinegar. Serve right away.

NOTE: For this recipe, the oil you choose will have a big impact on the flavour, as it is not just the oil for the salad dressing, but rather a major ingredient. I use either a fruity extra virgin olive oil or a cold-pressed canola oil that has a grassy tone. Both work brilliantly here.

1 SERVING = ½ THE RECIPE AS A LIGHT MAIN
PER SERVING: 380 CALORIES, 27 G TOTAL FAT, 8.6 G SATURATED FAT, 0 G TRANS FAT, 38 MG CHOLESTEROL, 404 MG SODIUM, 28.6 G CARBOHYDRATE, 6.4 G FIBRE, 22.6 G SUGARS, 0 G ADDED SUGARS, 11 G PROTEIN, 709 MG POTASSIUM
CARBOHYDRATE CHOICE = 1½ CHOICES

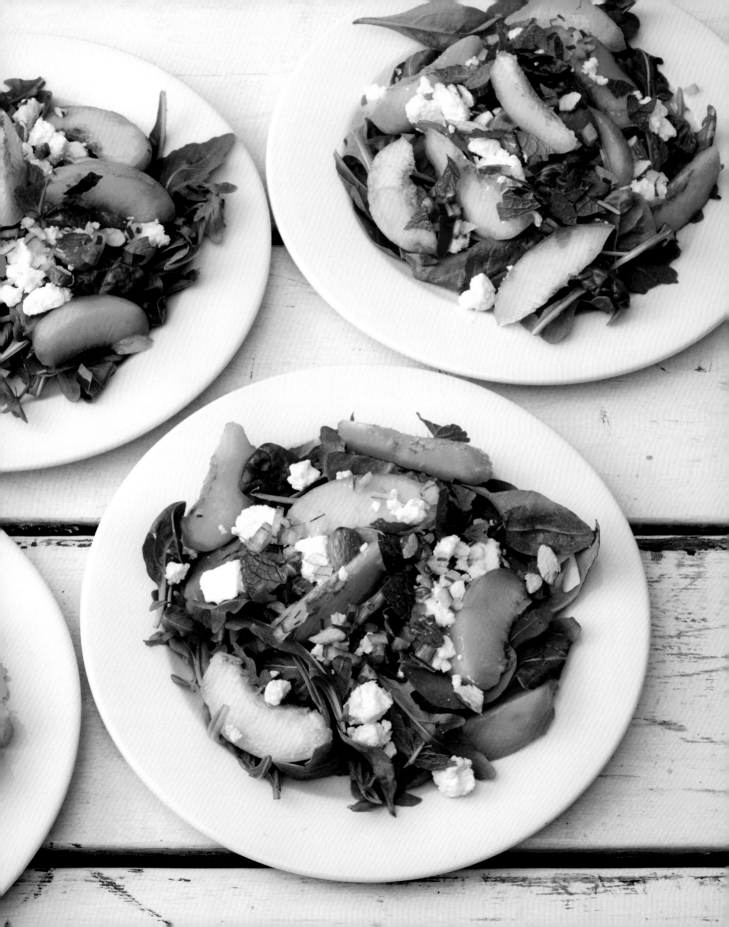

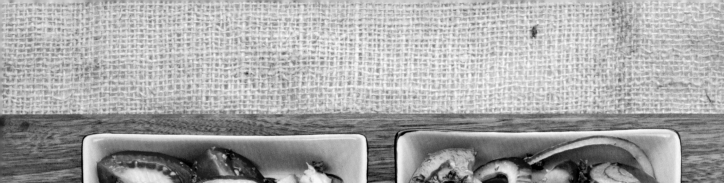
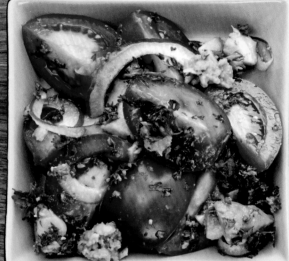
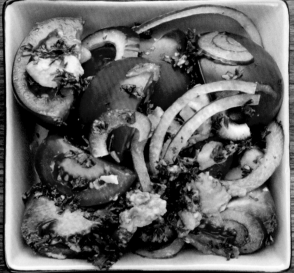
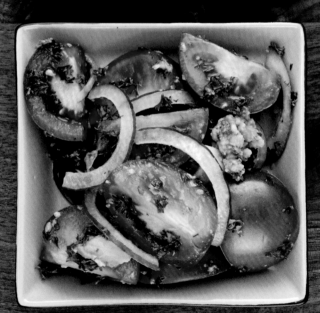
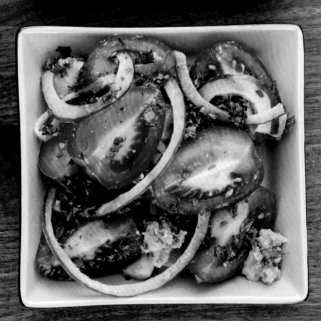

Tomato & Parsley Salad VEG V LF GF · *Serves 4 as a side*

I LOVE ENTERTAINING ALFRESCO DURING THE SUMMER MONTHS, and my perfect menu is one that reflects the season. In late July, when tomato season hits its peak, we eat our fill. Our friend Pete is a tomato connoisseur. Whenever he and his lovely wife, Mary, come to dinner, I make sure to serve an amazing tomato dish. Pete gave this a 5/5 tomato rating as the best tomato salad he had ever had. From his lips to your ears.

1 cup finely chopped fresh parsley leaves

½ cup thinly sliced red onion, in half moons

2 Tbsp fresh lemon juice

¼ tsp table salt

1 large ripe avocado

12 Campari or 9 Kumato tomatoes, quartered (see note)

1. In a large bowl, gently toss together the parsley, red onion, lemon juice, and salt.

2. Cut the avocado in half and remove the pit. Using a small spoon, scoop out small pieces of the avocado into the bowl.

3. Add the tomatoes, gently toss, and serve right away.

NOTE: If you can't find sweet Campari or Kumato tomatoes at your local grocery store, use cocktail tomatoes instead.

1 SERVING = 1 HEAPING CUP
PER SERVING: 111 CALORIES, 7.4 G TOTAL FAT, 1.1 G SATURATED FAT, 0 G TRANS FAT, 0 MG CHOLESTEROL, 151 MG SODIUM, 11.9 G CARBOHYDRATE, 5.2 G FIBRE, 4.9 G SUGARS, 0 G ADDED SUGARS, 2.2 G PROTEIN, 613 MG POTASSIUM
CARBOHYDRATE CHOICE = ½ CHOICE

Halloween Salad VEG GF · *Serves 5 as a side*

I MAY HAVE COME BY MY LOVE OF POMEGRANATES through my grandmother's roots. Gran, born in South Africa, was raised on the ruby red seeds, a.k.a. arils. She and her sisters would crush them and use the red liquid as rouge or lipstick. Every Halloween, Gran gave my siblings and me a pomegranate as a treat. One taste of those sweet and crunchy red seeds and a food memory was born. Halloween may conjure up food memories like pumpkins and candy apples for most people, but for me, it's all about Gran and pomegranates.

4 cups finely sliced green cabbage or a combo of red and green

2 cups chopped fresh parsley, leaves and stems

¾ cup finely sliced red onion

2 Tbsp cold-pressed canola oil or extra virgin olive oil

3 Tbsp apple cider vinegar

1 large pomegranate (see page 15)

1 cup (6 oz/170 g) crumbled feta cheese

6 Tbsp raw green pumpkin seeds

*

PROFESSIONAL HOME ECONOMIST TIP: When picking a pomegranate, look for weight, not colour. The heavier the pomegranate, the juicier it will be. Store a pomegranate for up to 1 month on the counter or up to 2 months in the fridge.

1. In a large bowl, toss together the cabbage, parsley, and red onion. Add the oil and vinegar and toss to combine. Place the bowl into your clean, empty kitchen sink. (I've totally got your attention, don't I?)

2. Find a heavy wooden spoon or a meat mallet. Cut the pomegranate in half. Take yourself and the cut pomegranate over to the sink. Working over the bowl of salad, gently place your thumbs on the outside stem of the half pomegranate, then press down and out. You're trying to crack it open just a bit. Place your hand under the cut side of the pomegranate and, using the heavy wooden spoon, start *whacking* the pomegranate on the pink peel side. It's fun and therapeutic all at the same time. Those wee seeds will fly onto the salad and hopefully not onto you, your counter, or your walls. Putting the bowl inside the sink helps with this. Repeat with the other half. Remove any white membrane that might have made it into the bowl. And voilà! You should have all the pomegranate seeds in the bowl now. See page 15 for a picture.

3. Wipe your hands and remove the bowl from the sink.

4. Add the feta cheese and toss the salad together. Divide into bowls and sprinkle each serving with an equal portion of pumpkin seeds.

1 SERVING = 2 CUPS
PER SERVING: 271 CALORIES, 18.6 G TOTAL FAT, 6.2 G SATURATED FAT, 0 G TRANS FAT,
28 MG CHOLESTEROL, 318 MG SODIUM, 19.5 G CARBOHYDRATE, 5 G FIBRE, 11.9 G SUGARS,
0 G ADDED SUGARS, 10.3 G PROTEIN, 461 MG POTASSIUM
CARBOHYDRATE CHOICE = 1 CHOICE

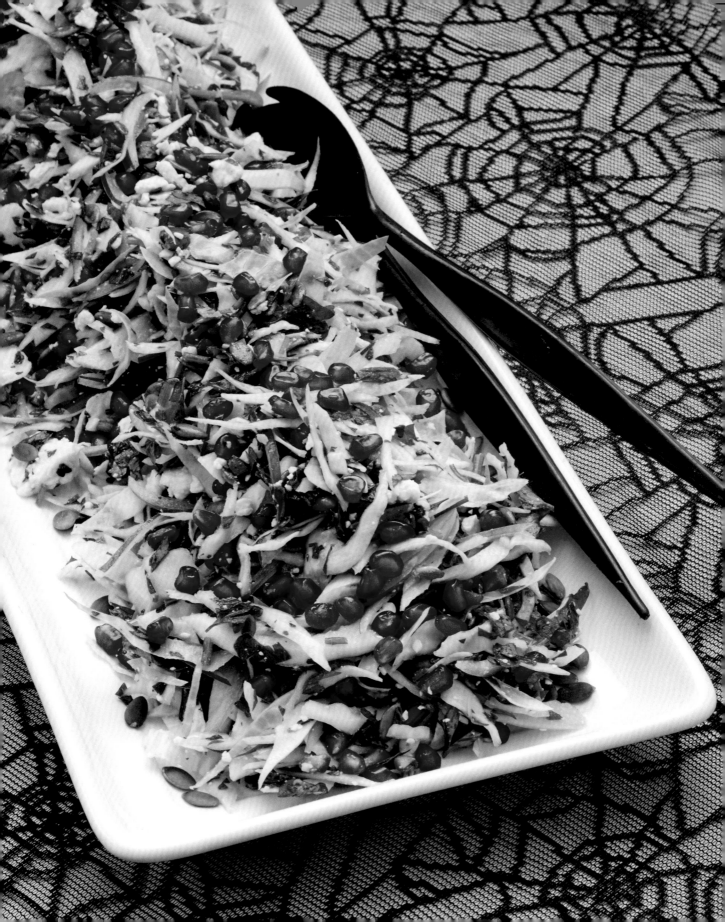

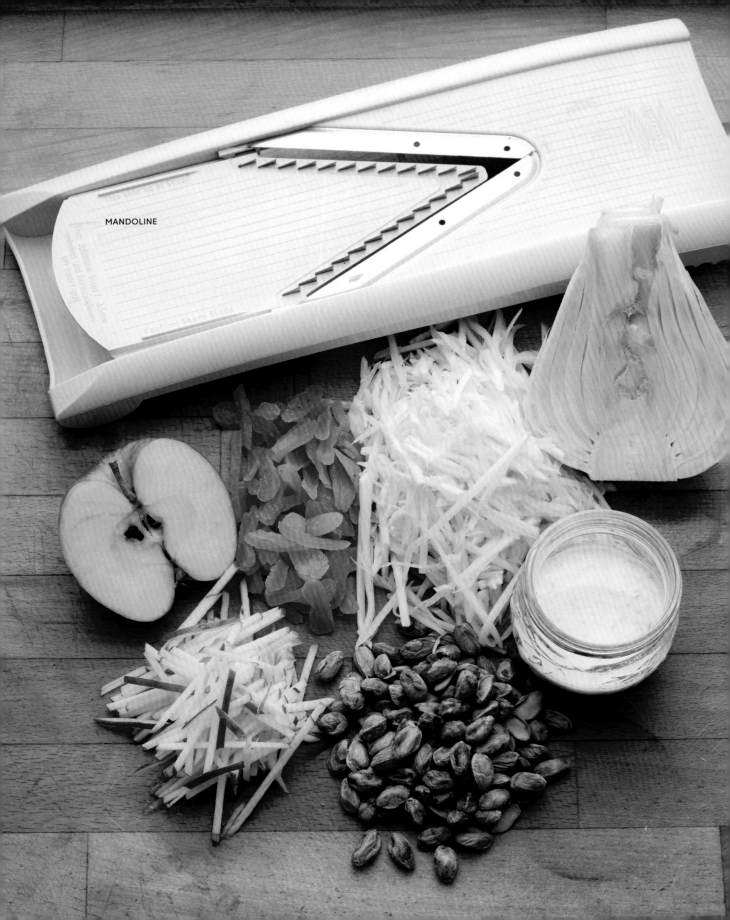

Springtime Apple & Fennel Slaw with Dried Apricots & Pistachios

VEG LF · *Serves 6 as a side*

A LITTLE CRUNCHY, A LITTLE SWEET, AND A LITTLE SALTY, this slaw holds the formula for all good relationships. And if you substitute "exciting" for "crunchy," this could be the formula for a good marriage, too.

SALAD DRESSING

2 Tbsp low-fat mayo

3 Tbsp fresh lime juice

1 tsp liquid honey

SLAW

3½ cups julienned fennel
(about 1 medium bulb)
(see note)

3 cups julienned apple
(I use 1 large Granny Smith
in the spring and 1 large
Honeycrisp in the summer)

½ cup thinly sliced dried apricots

¾ cup lightly salted shelled
whole pistachios

Zest of 1 lime

1. Make the salad dressing. In a large bowl, whisk together the mayo, lime juice, and honey until the honey has dissolved and the dressing is smooth.

2. Add the fennel, apple, and dried apricots and toss well. Set aside in the fridge for at least 1 hour and up to 3 hours to develop the flavours. Just before serving, add the pistachios and lime zest, toss, and serve.

NOTE: Julienning fruits and vegetables can absolutely be done by hand, but it's also a great opportunity to use a mandoline slicer. The different blades can be adjusted to get exactly the cuts you want, and all your pieces will come out looking exactly the same.

1 SERVING = 1 CUP
PER SERVING: 162 CALORIES, 8.3 G TOTAL FAT, 1.1 G SATURATED FAT, 0 G TRANS FAT,
1 MG CHOLESTEROL, 63 MG SODIUM, 20.7 G CARBOHYDRATE, 4.6 G FIBRE, 13.5 G SUGARS,
2.6 G ADDED SUGARS, 4 G PROTEIN, 457 MG POTASSIUM
CARBOHYDRATE CHOICE = 1 CHOICE

Summertime Asian-Style Coleslaw VEG V LF GF · *Serves 12 as a side*

I HAVE TRIED TO LOVE KIMCHI. I have tried many different versions made by many different chefs. I know it's a fermented food and a wonderful thing to eat for long-term health, but I have not found a recipe that spins my wheels. The funny thing is, I like the essence of kimchi. I love cabbage, ginger, garlic, radishes, green onions, and red pepper flakes. All those ingredients seem like they are meant to be together, so I created a kimchi-esque slaw in an East-meets-Mairlyn sort of way.

SALAD DRESSING

3 Tbsp lower-sodium or lite tamari

Zest of 1 lime

3 Tbsp fresh lime juice

1 Tbsp finely grated fresh ginger

2 tsp sesame oil

4 cloves garlic, minced

⅛ tsp red pepper flakes

SLAW

5 cups thinly sliced Savoy cabbage

1 orange pepper, julienned

6 radishes, julienned

3 green onions, whites included, thinly sliced

2 Tbsp chopped fresh cilantro leaves

2 Tbsp finely sliced fresh mint leaves

1. Make the salad dressing. In a large bowl, whisk together the tamari, lime zest, lime juice, ginger, oil, garlic, and red pepper flakes.

2. Add the cabbage, pepper, radishes, green onions, cilantro, and mint, and mix to combine. Set aside in the fridge for at least 1 hour and up to 3 hours to develop the flavours. Serve.

1 SERVING = ½ CUP
PER SERVING: 54 CALORIES, 1.7 G TOTAL FAT, 0.2 G SATURATED FAT, 0 G TRANS FAT, 0 MG CHOLESTEROL, 372 MG SODIUM, 8.3 G CARBOHYDRATE, 2.5 G FIBRE, 1.9 G SUGARS, 0 G ADDED SUGARS, 2.8 G PROTEIN, 271 MG POTASSIUM
CARBOHYDRATE CHOICE = < 1 CHOICE

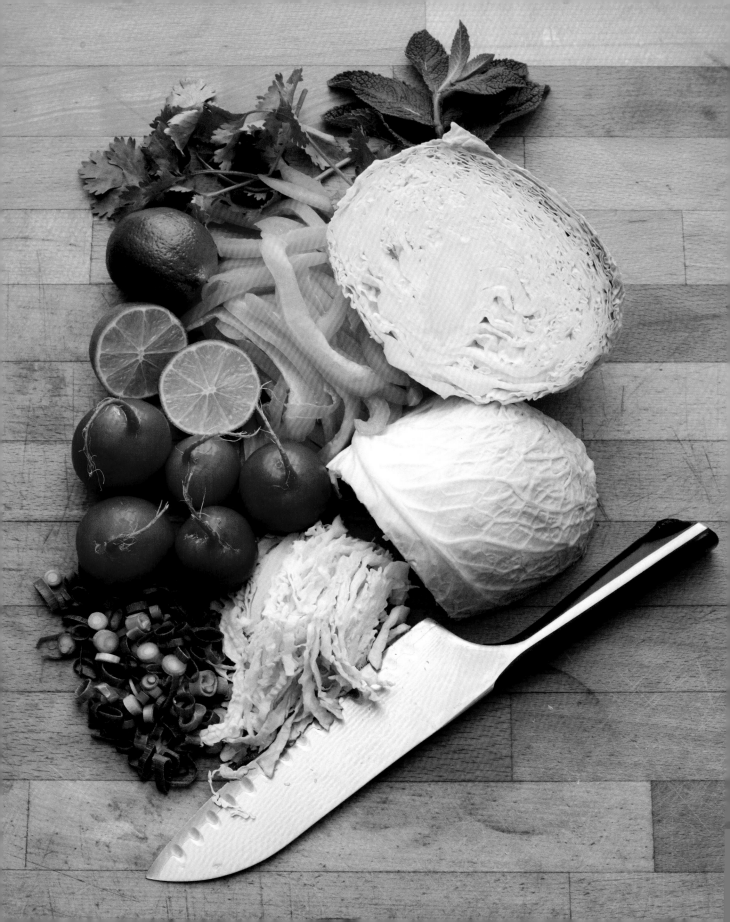

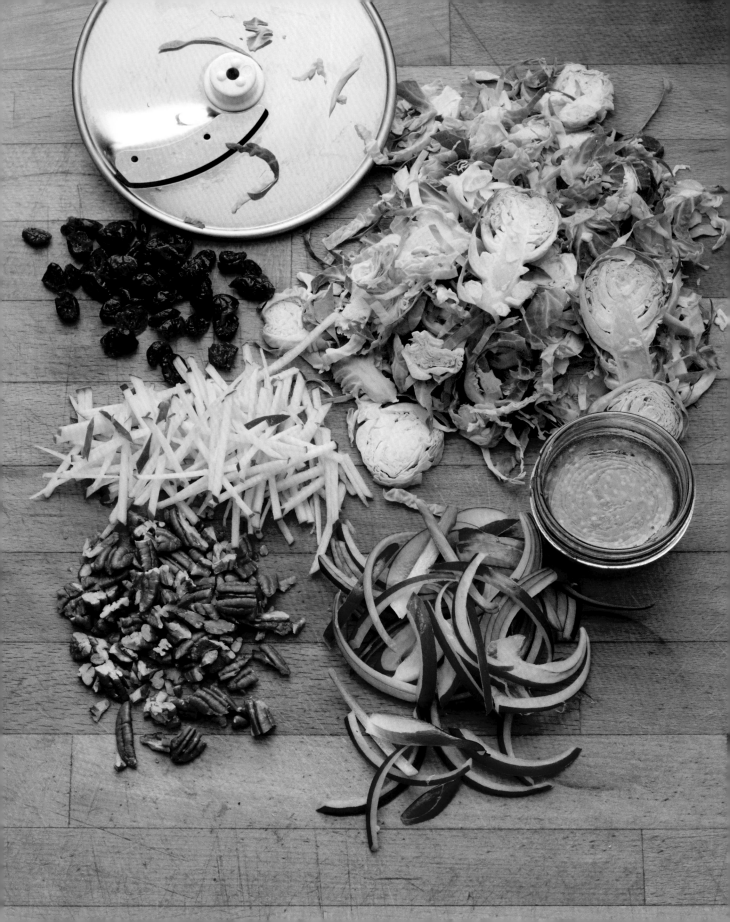

Fall Brussels Sprouts Slaw   VEG LF GF · *Serves 14 to 16 as a side*

IN MY VIGILANT QUEST TO ENCOURAGE EVERYONE to love cruciferous vegetables, specifically Brussels sprouts, I've come up with yet another incarnation of the basic slaw. Serve this at Thanksgiving when the wee cabbages (a.k.a. Brussels sprouts) are in season. Choose small, compact Brussels sprouts and eat them as soon as possible. The longer they hole up in your fridge, the stronger their flavour.

SALAD DRESSING

2 Tbsp canola oil

¼ cup apple cider vinegar

1 Tbsp liquid honey

1 Tbsp grainy Dijon mustard

SLAW

3½ cups (13 oz/370 g) whole Brussels sprouts

1 cup thinly sliced red onion

3 cups julienned Honeycrisp apple (about 1 large)

1 cup dried cranberries

1 cup pecans, coarsely chopped

1. Make the salad dressing. In a large bowl, whisk together the oil, vinegar, honey, and Dijon until the honey has dissolved.

2. Using a food processor fitted with the thin slicing blade, slice the Brussels sprouts.

3. Add the Brussels sprouts, red onion, apples, and dried cranberries to the bowl with the dressing. Set aside in the fridge for at least 1 hour and up to 3 hours to develop the flavours. Just before serving, add the pecans.

NOTE: This salad tends to wilt a bit the longer it's left. You'll get 8 cups if you eat it after 1 hour of rest, and 7 cups if you eat it after 3 hours—oh, that dreaded shrinkage.

1 SERVING = ½ CUP
PER SERVING: 116 CALORIES, 7.2 G TOTAL FAT, 0.6 G SATURATED FAT, 0 G TRANS FAT, 0 MG CHOLESTEROL, 20 MG SODIUM, 13.1 G CARBOHYDRATE, 2.8 G FIBRE, 7.9 G SUGARS, 4.9 G ADDED SUGARS, 2.1 G PROTEIN, 161 MG POTASSIUM
CARBOHYDRATE CHOICE = ½ CHOICE

Wintertime Kale Slaw   VEG LF · *Serves 4 as a side*

A VERY POPULAR BRUSSELS SPROUTS SLAW IS AVAILABLE in most large grocery stores. It's a clever idea that I decided to expand on. I switched out the Brussels sprouts and used more readily available kale, created a less sweet, slightly tangy dressing, added avocado as a heart-healthy fat, and, for colour plus an extra bang of nutrients, added red onions and peppers, creating a whole new taste experience. I'd say that gets an A+ from the healthy-eating gods.

SALAD DRESSING

2 Tbsp low-fat mayo

2 Tbsp apple cider vinegar

1 Tbsp pure amber maple syrup

SLAW

4 cups thinly sliced Tuscan kale, stalks removed (about ½ head)

1 large orange or yellow pepper, julienned

¼ cup thinly sliced red onion

1 perfectly ripe avocado

¼ cup dried cranberries

¼ cup unsalted raw green pumpkin seeds

*

PROFESSIONAL HOME ECONOMIST TIP: Turn this into a light vegetarian main course. Add 1 cup (6 oz/170 g) crumbled feta cheese and one large grapefruit, peeled and cut into small pieces. Toss well and serve.

1. Make the salad dressing. In a large bowl, whisk together the mayo, vinegar, and maple syrup.

2. Add the kale, pepper, and red onion and toss well.

3. Cut the avocado in half and remove the pit. Using a spoon, scoop out small pieces and add to the salad. Toss together well, sprinkle with cranberries and pumpkin seeds, and serve.

1 SERVING = 1¾ CUPS
PER SERVING: 229 CALORIES, 13.4 G TOTAL FAT, 2.1 G SATURATED FAT, 0 G TRANS FAT, 1 MG CHOLESTEROL, 93 MG SODIUM, 25.6 G CARBOHYDRATE, 6.4 G FIBRE, 12.8 G SUGARS, 8.1 G ADDED SUGARS, 4.4 G PROTEIN, 736 MG POTASSIUM
CARBOHYDRATE CHOICE = 1 CHOICE

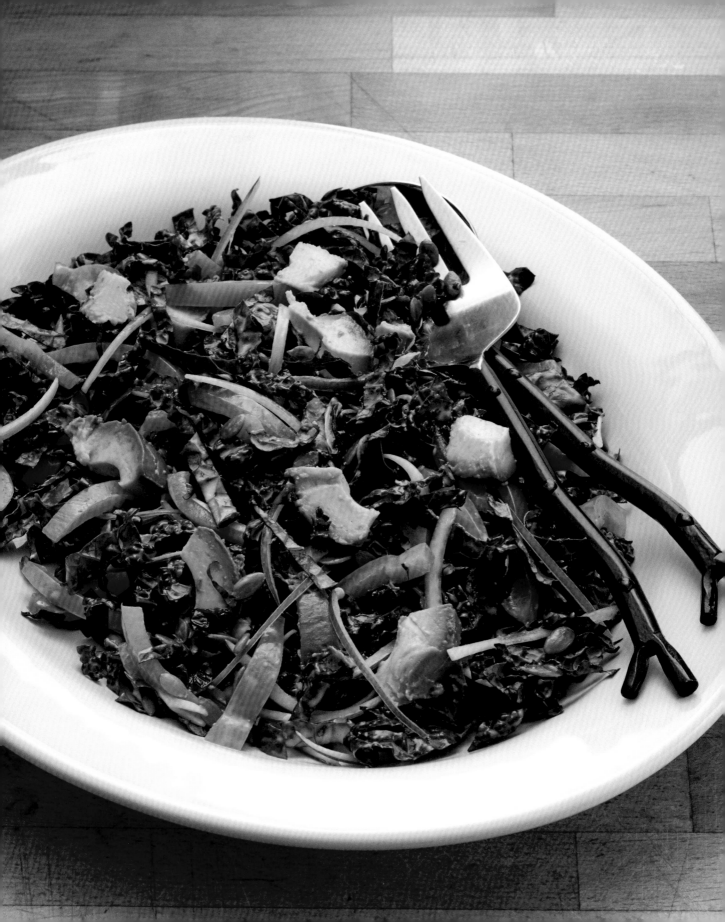

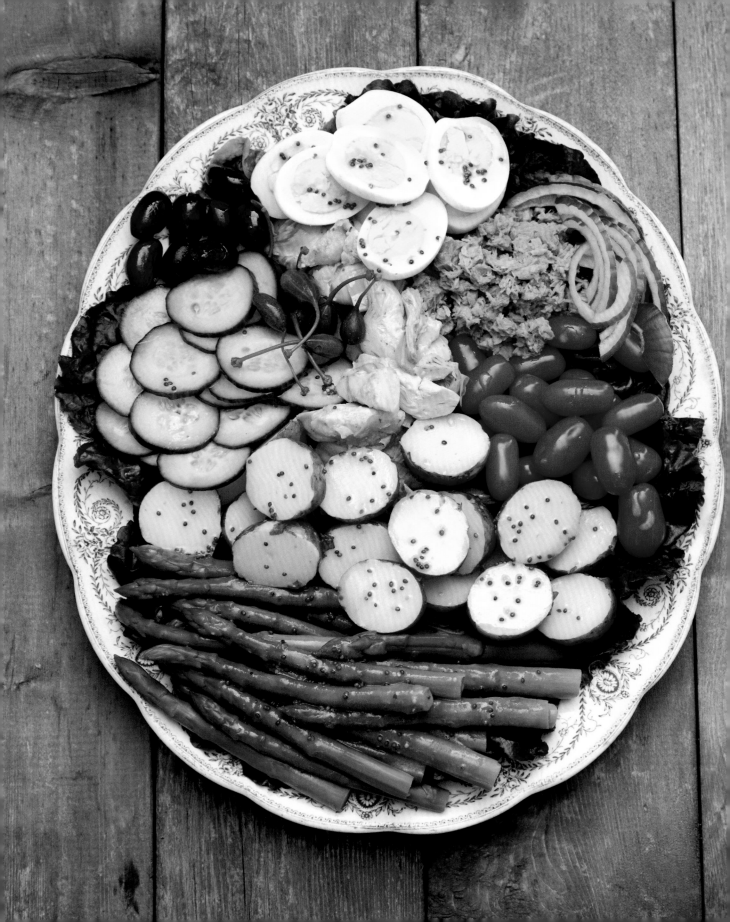

Nicoise Salad Platter LF GF · *Serves 4 as a main*

I MAKE THIS DINNER WHEN I HAVE LEFTOVER COOKED POTATOES, asparagus, and hard-cooked eggs in my fridge. What? Doesn't everyone have leftover potatoes, asparagus, and eggs in their fridge? Is it just me? Okay, but you can still make it if you cook the potatoes, asparagus, and eggs the day before. And just to entice you to have those lovely leftovers, this is the easiest dinner to serve during hot summer months. Assemble the salad the day of, serve with a bottle of crisp white wine and some fabulous bread, and sit back and enjoy your company.

SALAD

1 head red-tipped Bibb, Boston, or red leaf lettuce

12 mini potatoes, skin on, cooked, chilled, and halved

½ lb (225 g) cooked, chilled asparagus or green beans

4 omega-3 hard-cooked eggs, peeled and halved

1 (6 oz/170 g) can solid light tuna packed in oil or water, well drained

1 cup whole grape tomatoes

½ English cucumber, thinly sliced

8 Kalamata olives, pitted

8 caperberries (see note)

1 (6 fl oz/170 mL) jar marinated artichoke hearts, drained

¼ cup thinly sliced red onion

SALAD DRESSING

2 Tbsp fresh lemon juice

2 Tbsp extra virgin olive oil

1 Tbsp grainy Dijon mustard

2 tsp pure amber maple syrup

1. Rinse and pat dry the lettuce. Arrange the lettuce leaves so that they cover the bottom of a large platter.

2. Using the photo on the opposite page as your guide, arrange the potatoes, asparagus or green beans, eggs, tuna, tomatoes, cucumbers, olives, caperberries, artichoke hearts, and red onion over the lettuce leaves.

3. Make the salad dressing. Place the lemon juice, oil, Dijon, and maple syrup in a small glass jar with a tight-fitting lid and shake well. Drizzle the dressing equally over the salad ingredients and serve with a large fork and spoon so guests can help themselves.

NOTE: Caperberries are related to capers, which are the flower buds of the same bush. They're elongated and look like a skinny grape, and are less salty and have a more olive-like flavour. Most caperberries are hand-picked in midsummer and are naturally fermented to preserve their delicate texture, green colour, and unique flavour.

1 SERVING = ¼ OF THE PLATTER
PER SERVING: 366 CALORIES, 20.6 G TOTAL FAT, 3.9 G SATURATED FAT, 0 G TRANS FAT, 76 MG CHOLESTEROL, 629 MG SODIUM, 30.4 G CARBOHYDRATE, 4.6 G FIBRE, 5.2 G SUGARS, 1 G ADDED SUGARS, 20.3 G PROTEIN, 1084 MG POTASSIUM
CARBOHYDRATE CHOICE = 2 CHOICES

Chickpea & Tabbouleh Salad with Roasted Grape Tomatoes

VEG V LF GF · *Serves 4 or 5 as a side*

SEVERAL YEARS AGO, ONE OF MY NEIGHBOURS GAVE ME all her old copies of *Martha Stewart Living* magazine. I sat on my front porch that summer tearing out recipes and getting inspired. Martha schooled an entire generation on everything from how to brighten your laundry to stencilling leaves on lampshades. Sadly, I've never had the patience for crafts, but the pictures of the food? That was a whole other ballpark. This recipe was inspired by one of Martha's pictures.

¾ cup quinoa

4 cups grape tomatoes, halved

10 cloves garlic, chopped

1 Tbsp canola oil

1 Tbsp balsamic vinegar

Zest and juice of 2 large lemons

2 Tbsp extra virgin olive oil

2 cups finely chopped fresh parsley leaves

1 cup julienned fresh mint leaves

1 cup diced red onion

1 (19 fl oz/540 mL) can no-salt-added chickpeas, rinsed and well drained

½ tsp table salt

1 SERVING = 1½ CUPS
PER SERVING: 357 CALORIES, 13.4 G TOTAL FAT, 1.6 G SATURATED FAT, 0 G TRANS FAT, 0 MG CHOLESTEROL, 302 MG SODIUM, 50.4 G CARBOHYDRATE, 8.8 G FIBRE, 6.1 G SUGARS, 0 G ADDED SUGARS, 11.6 G PROTEIN, 829 MG POTASSIUM
CARBOHYDRATE CHOICE = 3 CHOICES

1. The night before or at least 4 hours before serving, prepare the quinoa. In a fine-mesh strainer, rinse the quinoa under cold running water. Transfer the quinoa to a 2½-quart saucepan, add 1½ cups water, and bring to a boil. Cover, reduce heat to low, and simmer for 10 to 14 minutes, until all the liquid has been absorbed and the quinoa is light and fluffy. Remove the pot from the heat, fluff the quinoa with a fork, cover, and let sit for 10 minutes. Place the quinoa in a container with a tight-fitting lid and refrigerate until you are ready to make the salad.

2. Preheat the oven to 425°F. Line a 9 × 13-inch metal baking dish with wet parchment paper (see page 15).

3. Place the tomatoes, garlic, canola oil, and vinegar in the pan and lightly mix using a fork. Roast in the oven for 35 to 40 minutes, until the tomatoes are soft and the peels are starting to caramelize. Remove from the oven and let cool on a wire rack for about 40 minutes, until the tomatoes are at room temperature. The tomatoes can also be prepared a day in advance and kept refrigerated in a container with a tight-fitting lid until you're ready.

4. To make the salad, whisk the lemon zest, lemon juice, and olive oil in a large bowl. Add the roasted tomatoes, parsley, mint, and red onion. Mix well.

5. Add the quinoa, drained chickpeas, and salt. Stir to combine and refrigerate for at least 2 hours and up to 6 hours before serving.

NOTE: Most tabbouleh recipes use bulgur wheat or couscous. I decided years ago, as a salute to all my friends who have celiac disease, that I would forever make my tabbouleh with quinoa, making it a gluten-free dish everyone will love.

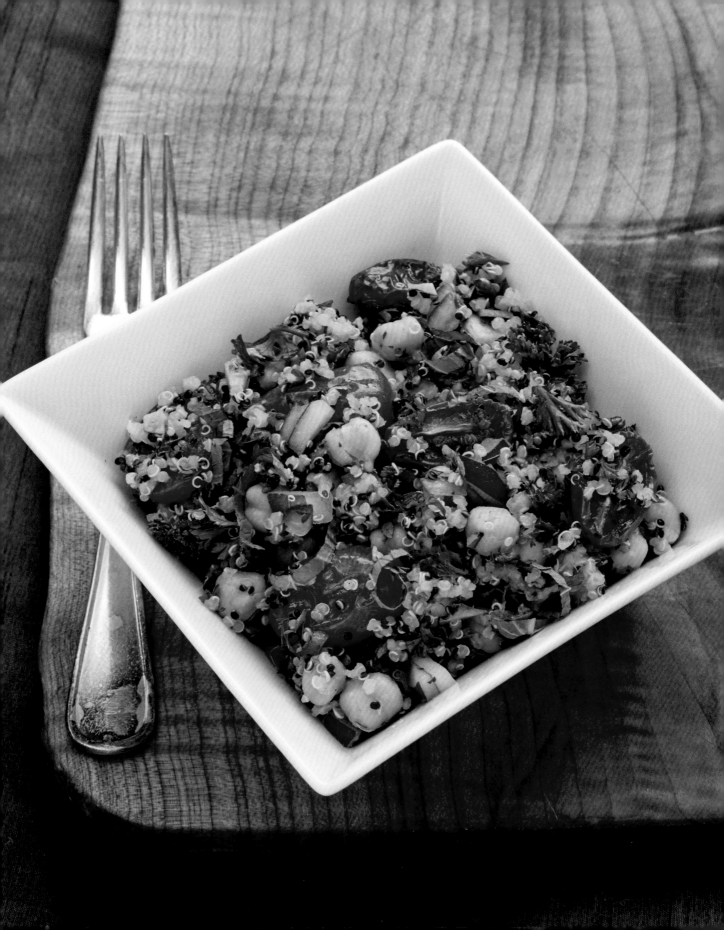

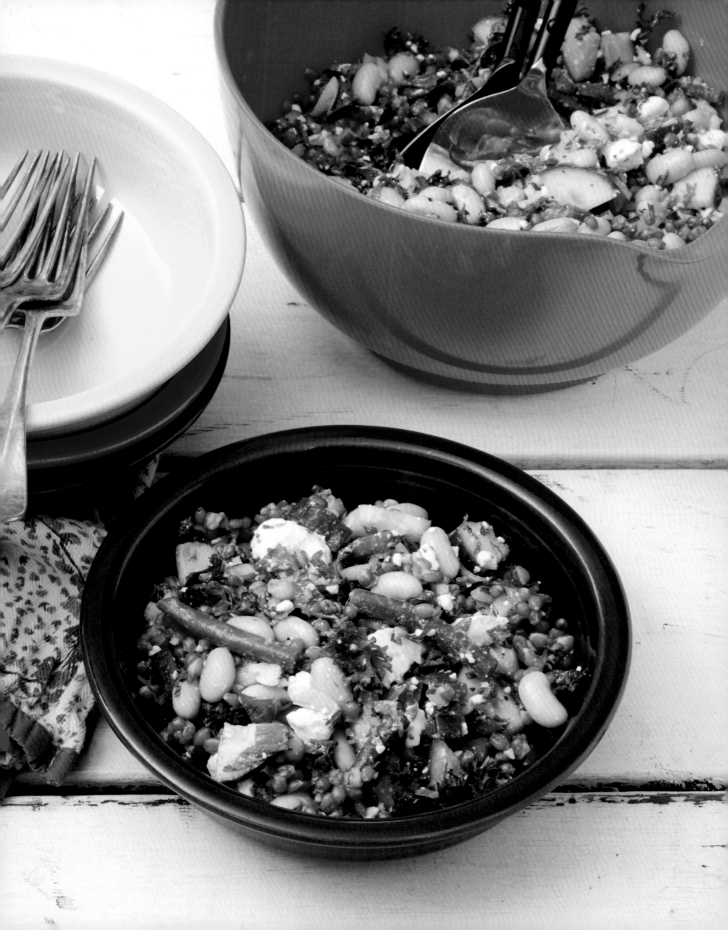

Fatoush   VEG · *Serves 4 as a side*

MOST CULTURES HAVE RECIPES THAT USE LEFTOVER CARBS. Fatoush is a Lebanese salad that uses stale pita bread tossed with cucumbers, parsley, mint, feta, and onions. In the Mairlyn-ized version of fatoush, I use cooked wheat berries instead of pita bread, going right to the heart of any bread recipe and using the whole wheat kernels.

SALAD

¾ cup (4 oz/118 g) green beans

1 cup tightly packed fresh parsley leaves

1 cup tightly packed fresh mint leaves

1 (19 fl oz/540 mL) can no-salt-added white kidney beans, rinsed and well drained

½ English cucumber, quartered and chopped into ½-inch pieces

⅓ cup diced red onion

1 cup cooked wheat berries (see page 13)

½ cup (3 oz/85 g) crumbled feta cheese

SALAD DRESSING

Zest of 1 large lemon

3 Tbsp fresh lemon juice

3 Tbsp extra virgin olive oil

1 large clove garlic, crushed

½ tsp freshly ground black pepper

⅛ tsp table salt

1. Rinse and cut off the ends of the green beans. Place the beans in a small saucepan, barely cover with water, put on high heat, and bring to a boil. Boil for 1 minute, then immediately transfer the beans to a bowl of cold water to stop the cooking process. Drain the beans again and set aside.

2. Rinse the parsley and mint well and pat dry. You don't want the herbs to be wet when they go into the salad.

3. Make the salad dressing. In a large bowl, whisk together the lemon zest, lemon juice, oil, garlic, pepper, and salt.

4. Add the white kidney beans, cucumber, red onion, parsley, and mint and mix well.

5. Cut the green beans into 2-inch pieces and add to the salad. Add the cooked wheat berries, sprinkle with feta cheese, gently toss, and serve.

1 SERVING = 1¾ CUPS
PER SERVING: 368 CALORIES, 16 G TOTAL FAT, 4.6 G SATURATED FAT, 0 G TRANS FAT, 18 MG CHOLESTEROL, 262 MG SODIUM, 43 G CARBOHYDRATE, 10.6 G FIBRE, 3.3 G SUGARS, 0 G ADDED SUGARS, 15.9 G PROTEIN, 687 MG POTASSIUM
CARBOHYDRATE CHOICE = 2 CHOICES

Asian Spring Roll Salad   VEG V LF · *Serves 7 as a side*

FRESH VIETNAMESE SPRING ROLLS ARE FABULOUS TO EAT, and I order them almost every time I see them on a menu. While I was developing recipes for this book, I thought I'd put spring rolls in, but after making the 20th spring roll, chopping, dipping rice papers into warm water, patting them dry, stuffing them, and rolling them up, I decided that I never wanted to make another spring roll, ever. But what if I used the elements of the spring rolls and made a main course salad? Bingo! Goodbye rolling and hello fabulous main-course vegetarian salad with loads of flavour.

2 (12 oz/350 g) packages extra-firm tofu

DRESSING AND MARINADE

4 cloves garlic, minced

¼ cup lower-sodium or lite tamari

¼ cup natural rice vinegar

1 Tbsp wasabi paste

1 Tbsp sesame oil

3 Tbsp grated fresh ginger

Zest of 2 limes

¼ cup fresh lime juice

SALAD

8 oz (225 g) whole grain or whole grain plus protein spaghettini

3 ripe mangos, peeled and julienned

2 red peppers, julienned

6 green onions, whites included, thinly sliced

6 radishes, julienned

1 cup chopped fresh cilantro leaves

¼ cup thinly sliced fresh mint leaves

1. Drain the tofu and cut each block into ½-inch cubes. Set aside.

2. Make the dressing and marinade. In a medium bowl, whisk together the garlic, tamari, vinegar, wasabi paste, oil, ginger, lime zest, and lime juice. Pour half of it into a resealable plastic bag and reserve the rest.

3. Place the tofu into the plastic bag and seal, making sure that the marinade coats all the tofu. Refrigerate for at least 4 hours and up to 12 hours.

4. Break the spaghettini in half and cook according to the package directions. Drain well. Mix the drained pasta with the reserved dressing and transfer to a container with a tight-fitting lid. Refrigerate for at least 4 hours and up to 12 hours.

5. To make the salad, combine the mangos, peppers, green onions, radishes, cilantro, mint, and pasta in a very large bowl. Make sure to scrape out any extra dressing.

6. Add the marinated tofu and any of the marinade that wasn't absorbed. Gently toss together. Serve right away or refrigerate for up to 24 hours.

NOTE: Ataulfo mangos, sometimes called honey mangos, are my favourite variety. They have sweet, firm flesh without any fibres and have a whole lot of fruit on each seed pod. They are grown in Mexico, Ecuador, and Peru and are available from March to June.

1 SERVING = 2 CUPS
PER SERVING: 294 CALORIES, 5.1 G TOTAL FAT, 0.8 G SATURATED FAT, 0 G TRANS FAT, 0 MG CHOLESTEROL, 654 MG SODIUM, 44.7 G CARBOHYDRATE, 5.4 G FIBRE, 15.6 G SUGARS, 0 G ADDED SUGARS, 14.6 G PROTEIN, 426 MG POTASSIUM
CARBOHYDRATE CHOICE = 2½ CHOICES

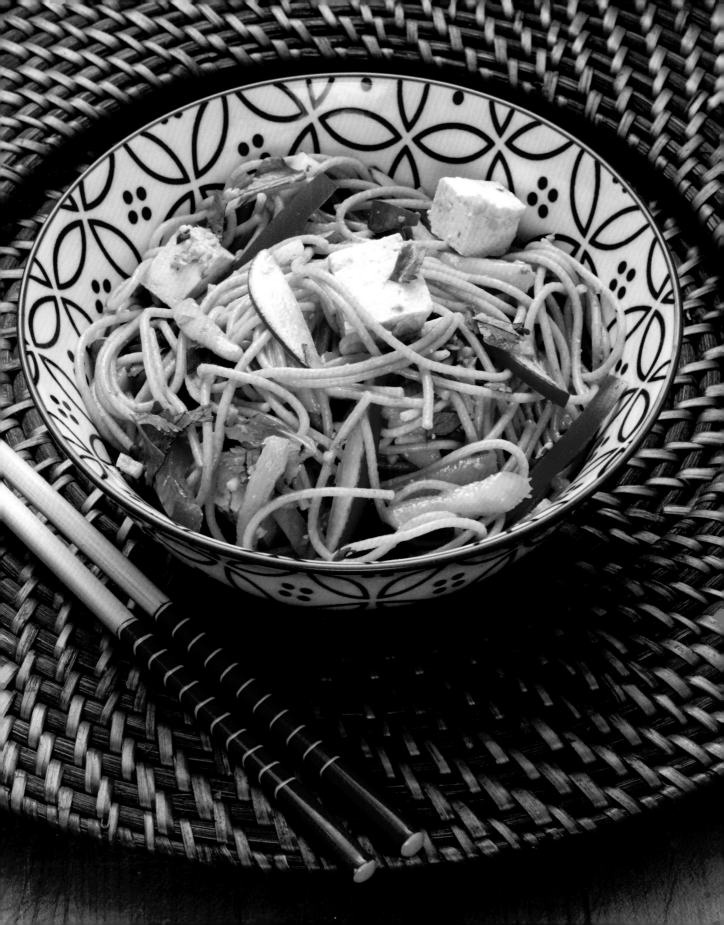

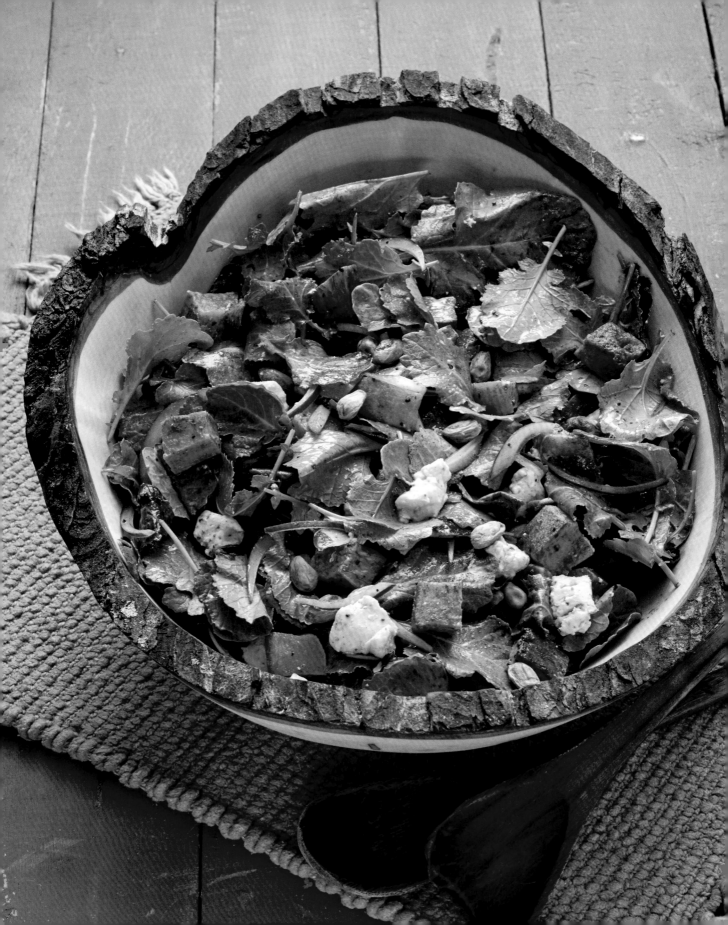

Roasted Squash & Kale Salad with Pistachios & Fig Goat Cheese

VEG GF · *Serves 4 as a side*

I DON'T LIKE TO WASTE FOOD, so I often find myself repurposing food from one recipe to use in another. Here, you can make the recipe for Oven-Roasted Butternut Squash (page 168) and reserve 2 cups of the cooked squash for this salad. Because the squash is already roasted, all you do is a bit of slicing and your dinner salad is ready.

SALAD DRESSING

2 Tbsp extra virgin olive oil or canola oil

2 Tbsp fresh lemon juice

1 tsp liquid honey

SALAD

4 cups baby kale, rinsed and dried

½ cup thinly sliced red onion

2 cups Oven-Roasted Butternut Squash (page 168)

2½ oz (70 g) fig goat cheese

½ cup roasted, lightly salted shelled whole pistachios

1. Make the salad dressing. In a large bowl, whisk together the oil, lemon juice, and honey.

2. Add the baby kale, red onion, and roasted squash and toss gently. Crumble the goat cheese into the bowl, mix well, and divide equally among four bowls. Sprinkle each bowl with 2 Tbsp pistachios. You can serve this as an appetizer salad or as a side to grilled chicken or fish.

1 SERVING = 1¼ CUPS
PER SERVING: 248 CALORIES, 15.9 G TOTAL FAT, 4.2 G SATURATED FAT, 0 G TRANS FAT, 0 MG CHOLESTEROL, 135 MG SODIUM, 23 G CARBOHYDRATE, 4.5 G FIBRE, 7.2 G SUGARS, 1.9 G ADDED SUGARS, 7.6 G PROTEIN, 461 MG POTASSIUM
CARBOHYDRATE CHOICE = 1 CHOICE

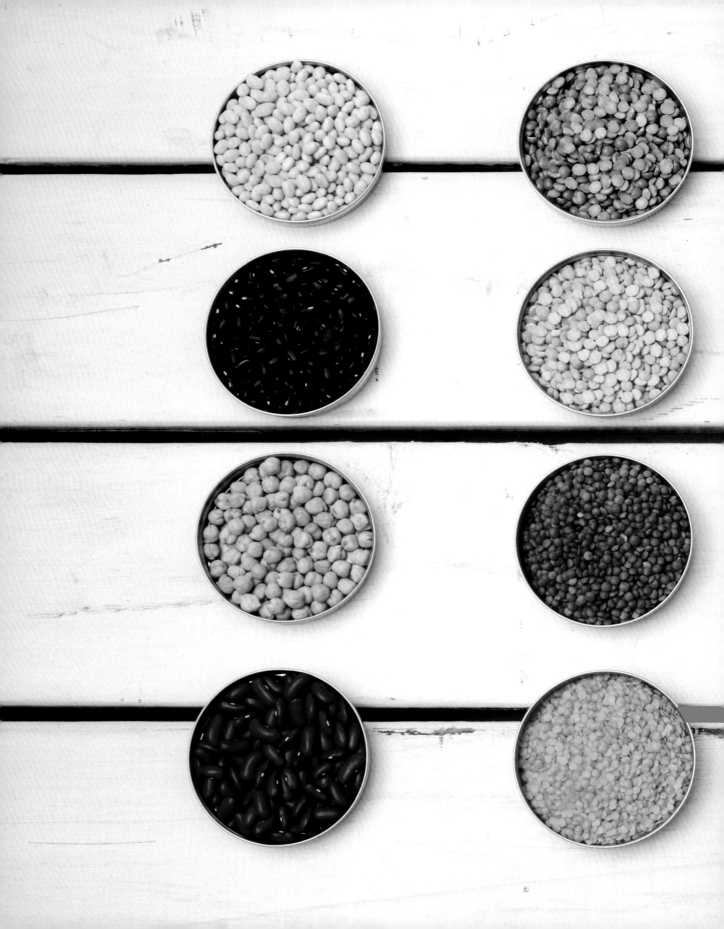

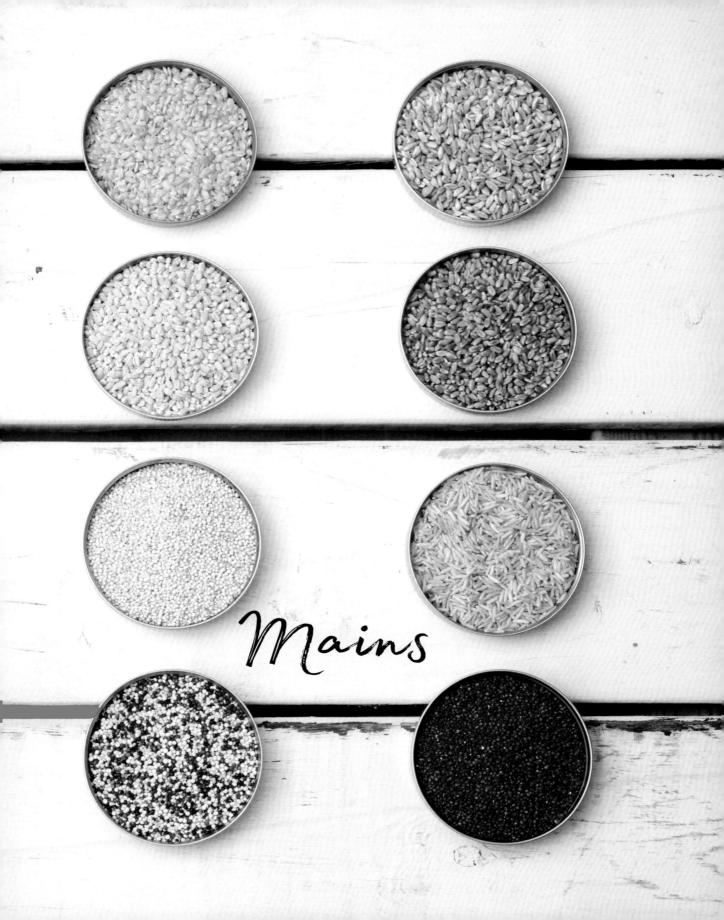

Mains

Ah, the Dinner Hour, sometimes known as the Witching Hour, the Hell Hour, or the I Don't Have a Clue What to Make for Dinner Tonight Hour.

Dinner doesn't have to be a nightmare for you or anyone else living under your roof. That doesn't mean the solution is calling for a large pizza or any other fast-food option. I've got some ideas in this chapter to help get you through.

1. Make friends with your kitchen. It might not be working for you because it isn't organized, the pantry isn't helping you, or you don't have a clue what you're going to make when you hit the kitchen at 5:57 p.m.

2. Plan out meals in advance. Sitting down on the weekend and planning what you are going to cook for the week may sound like a complete pain, but it will help you in the long run. When you walk in the door Tuesday night, you'll know you're going to make Skillet Enchiladas (page 150) and half the mealtime battle is solved.

3. Enlist your family to help prepare dinner. Once it's ready, sit down at the dinner table and make it a TV-, device-, and phone call–free zone. Connect with your family, talk about your day, and have a conversation. If this is new to you and your family, it's going to take time, especially if you have teens, but hang in there—it's worth it.

4. Every meal gives you another opportunity to add fibre to your day, and dinner is no exception. I have created some dinner options that range from the lower fibre stratosphere all the way to the top.

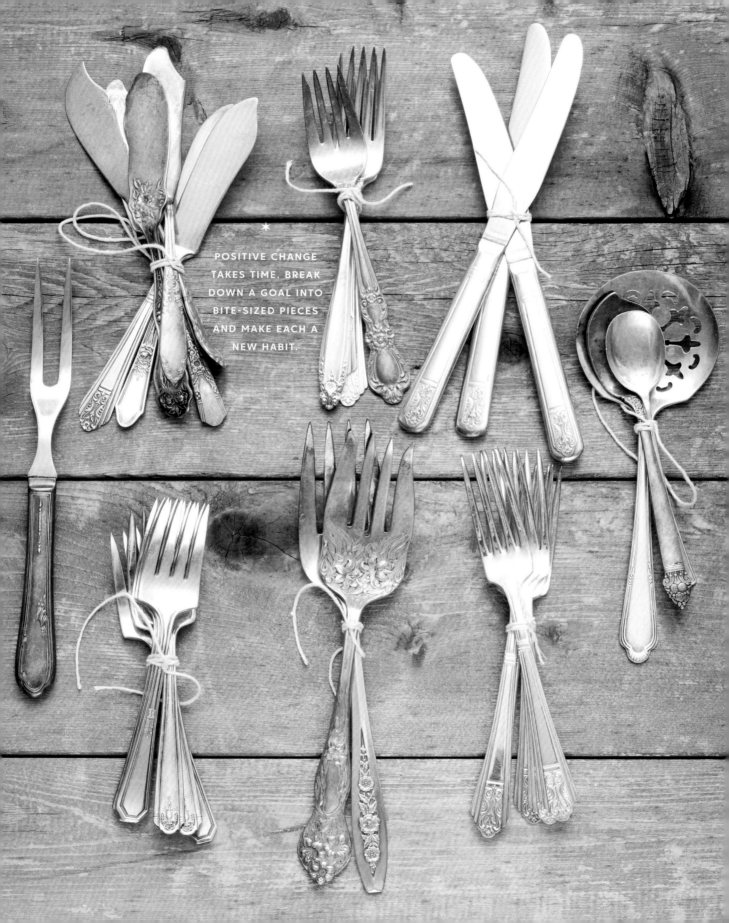

★

POSITIVE CHANGE
TAKES TIME. BREAK
DOWN A GOAL INTO
BITE-SIZED PIECES
AND MAKE EACH A
NEW HABIT.

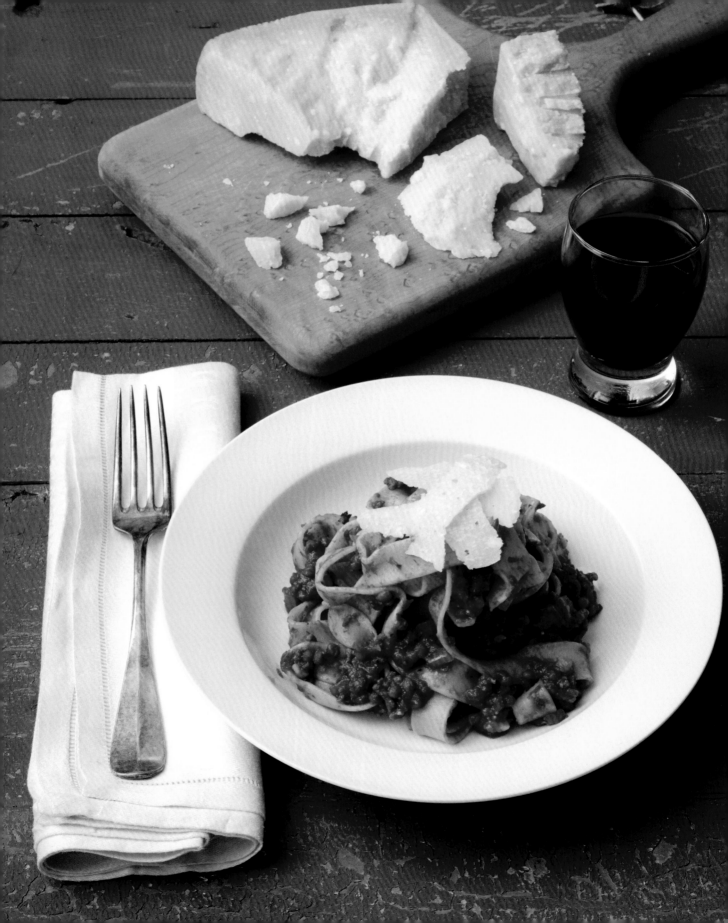

Big-Batch Bolognese Sauce *Makes 12 cups*

THIS THICK MEAT SAUCE IS A FABULOUS WAY to extend beef and add heart-healthy lentils to your diet at the same time. I like to freeze some leftover sauce for those hectic days when I get home and don't have a clue what I should make for dinner.

1¼ lb (560 g) extra-lean ground beef

2 onions, diced

8 cloves garlic, minced

1 Tbsp dried oregano leaves

1 tsp freshly ground black pepper

½ tsp table salt

2 (28 fl oz/796 mL) cans crushed or ground tomatoes

¼ cup balsamic vinegar

2 (19 fl oz/540 mL) cans lentils, rinsed and well drained

2 Mairlyn's Flavour Bombs (page 77) or ¼ cup store-bought pesto

1 (8.8 oz/250 g) package pappardelle pasta

WHEN SERVING OVER PASTA, EACH PORTION GETS:

1 Tbsp extra virgin olive oil

1 Tbsp shaved Parmigiano-Reggiano

1. Heat a Dutch oven or a large saucepan with high sides over medium heat. Add the beef, breaking it up into small pieces as it browns.

2. Add the onions and garlic and sauté for 3 to 5 minutes until the onions soften, but be careful not to burn the garlic.

3. Add the oregano, pepper, salt, tomatoes, balsamic vinegar, and lentils. Mix well. Bring to a simmer, cover, reduce heat to low, and cook, stirring occasionally, for 55 to 60 minutes.

4. Add the Flavour Bombs and let them melt (or pesto). Remove the sauce from the heat.

5. Cook the pasta according to the package instructions. Combine the cooked pasta with 4 cups sauce and gently combine.

6. Divide the pasta and sauce equally among four plates. Drizzle each with 1 Tbsp extra virgin olive oil and 1 Tbsp shaved Parmigiano-Reggiano. I always serve this fabulous dinner with red wine. The leftover sauce can be frozen for up to 3 months.

1 SERVING = 1 CUP BOLOGNESE SAUCE + ¼ OF A 8.8 OZ (250 G) PACKAGE OF PAPPARDELLE PASTA PER SERVING: 647 CALORIES, 26.9 G TOTAL FAT, 6.3 G SATURATED FAT, 0 G TRANS FAT, 98 MG CHOLESTEROL, 680 MG SODIUM, 72.5 G CARBOHYDRATE, 11.6 G FIBRE, 8.3 G SUGARS, 0 G ADDED SUGARS, 28.3 G PROTEIN, 865 MG POTASSIUM
CARBOHYDRATE CHOICE = 4 CHOICES

Black Beans & Rice LF GF · *Serves 7 as a main or 14 as a side*

COOKING DINNER WITH MY BFF MICHALE at her cottage is usually a sit-down affair for a crowd. We usually serve a protein, many vegetables, an enormous salad, and one bean dish for the bean lovers in the group (insert my name here!). This dish fits the bill: super-delicious and loaded with fibre.

2 Tbsp canola oil

3 onions, diced

8 cloves garlic, minced

1 orange pepper, coarsely chopped

1 yellow pepper, coarsely chopped

2 Tbsp smoked paprika

½ tsp freshly ground black pepper

¼ tsp table salt

1 (28 fl oz/796 mL) can no-salt-added chopped tomatoes

1½ cups brown basmati rice, rinsed well and drained

1 (19 fl oz/540 mL) can no-salt-added black beans, rinsed and well drained

½ cup lower-sodium vegetable broth

2 Tbsp pure amber maple syrup

1 Tbsp Worcestershire sauce

Hot sauce, for serving (optional)

1. Place a large Dutch oven over medium heat. Add the oil and onions and sauté until the onions start to brown, 4 to 6 minutes.

2. Add the garlic, both peppers, paprika, black pepper, and salt and sauté for 1 minute.

3. Add the tomatoes, rice, beans, broth, maple syrup, and Worcestershire sauce. Bring to a rapid boil. Cover, reduce heat to low, and simmer for 50 to 60 minutes, until the rice is tender.

4. Remove from heat, stir, and let sit, covered, for 10 minutes. Serve, adding hot sauce if desired. Store any leftovers in the fridge for up to 3 days.

1 SERVING = 1½ CUPS
PER SERVING: 319 CALORIES, 5.8 G TOTAL FAT, 0.4 G SATURATED FAT, 0 G TRANS FAT, 0 MG CHOLESTEROL, 102 MG SODIUM, 60.4 G CARBOHYDRATE, 10 G FIBRE, 11.9 G SUGARS, 3.3 G ADDED SUGARS, 12.7 G PROTEIN, 656 MG POTASSIUM
CARBOHYDRATE CHOICE = 3½ CHOICES

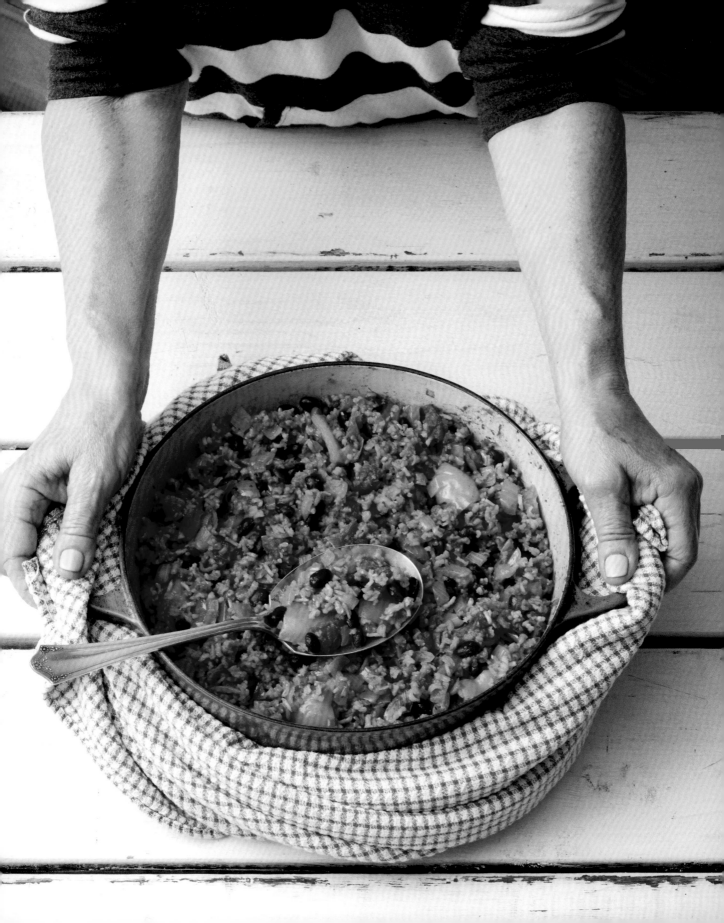

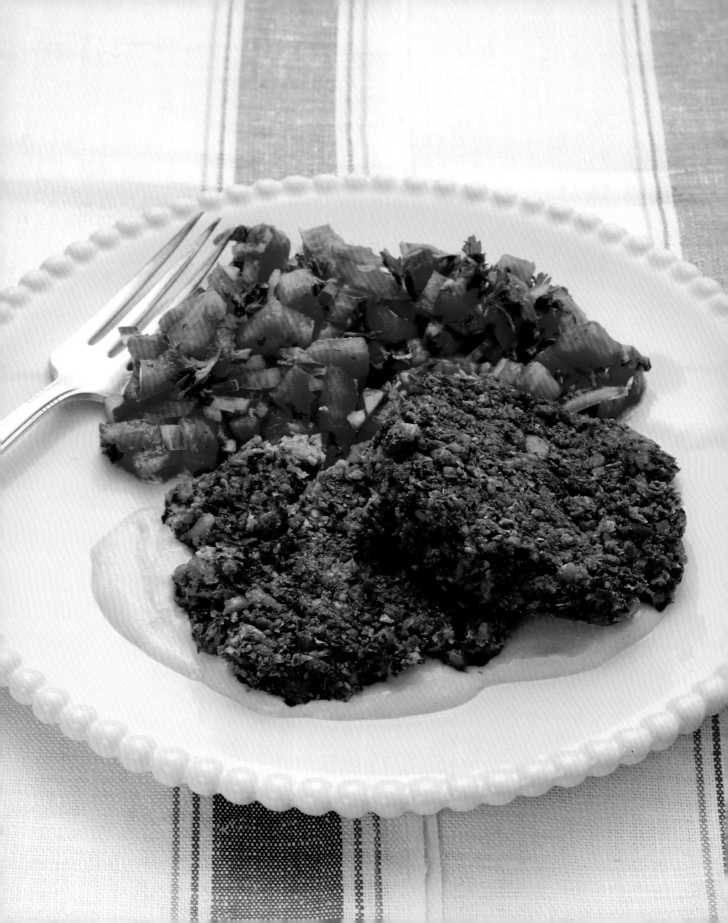

Pan-Fried Falafel with Tahini Sauce VEG V LF · *Serves 4*

THE PLACE: Vancouver.

THE YEAR: 1978.

THE PERSON: Me.

THE EVENT: The first time I tasted a falafel and experienced the extraordinary flavour explosion.

THE DIALOGUE: "WHAAATT is this and whatever it is, it's amazing! And, oh, shoot, it's deep-fried."

IT TOOK ME YEARS TO GET THIS RECIPE RIGHT, because no way was I going to be duped by a deep fat fryer. My version of falafel requires only a frying pan and a fraction of the oil. And best of all, it's made without losing any of those amazing Middle Eastern flavours.

1 (19 fl oz/540 mL) can no-salt-added chickpeas, rinsed and well drained

4 cloves garlic

¼ medium red onion, cut in chunks

1 cup well-packed fresh cilantro, leaves and stems

1 cup well-packed fresh parsley, leaves and stems

1 Tbsp ground cumin

2 tsp ground coriander

¼ tsp chili powder

¼ tsp table salt

¼ tsp freshly ground black pepper

4 Tbsp canola oil (divided)

¼ cup chickpea flour

TAHINI SAUCE

¼ cup tahini

2 Tbsp fresh lemon juice

2 tsp hot sauce

NOTE: One of my recipe testers, JC Chessell, makes these on a Sunday for lunches during the week. She just reheats the falafels, and lunch is ready.

1. Preheat the oven to 200°F and set up your food processor with the blade attachment. Line a baking sheet with parchment paper and set aside. Add the chickpeas to the food processor and pulse until they look crumbly, but not pasty. If you've hit pasty, you've gone too far. Transfer the chickpeas to a large bowl.

2. Add the garlic to the food processor and pulse until it is cut up into small pieces. Add the red onion, cilantro, and parsley. Pulse until finely chopped. Add to the bowl with the chickpeas and stir well. Add the cumin, coriander, chili powder, salt, and pepper to the bowl and stir well. Add 2 Tbsp canola oil, mix in, and sprinkle with the chickpea flour. Stir until the flour is well incorporated. Form into eight equal patties about ¼ cup each, and flatten them out to ½ inch thick.

3. Heat a large 12- or 14-inch non-stick skillet over medium-high heat. When the pan is hot, add 1 Tbsp oil and four patties. Fry the patties on each side until a deep brown, 8 to 10 minutes total. Transfer the cooked patties to the baking sheet and keep warm in the oven. Repeat with the remaining patties.

4. Meanwhile, make the sauce. Whisk together the tahini, 3 Tbsp water, lemon juice, and hot sauce in a small bowl.

5. Place a large dollop of tahini sauce on each plate and top with two falafel. Serve with diced tomatoes, parsley, and red onion as seen in the picture, or with Tomato & Parsley Salad (page 103).

1 SERVING = 2 FALAFEL + 2 GENEROUS TBSP TAHINI SAUCE
PER SERVING: 433 CALORIES, 24.6 G TOTAL FAT, 2.4 G SATURATED FAT, 0 G TRANS FAT,
0 MG CHOLESTEROL, 242 MG SODIUM, 31.7 G CARBOHYDRATE, 7 G FIBRE, 2.1 G SUGARS,
0 G ADDED SUGARS, 10.8 G PROTEIN, 389 MG POTASSIUM
CARBOHYDRATE CHOICE = 1½ CHOICES

Spicy Slow-Cooker Vegetarian Chili VEG · *Makes 12 cups*

THIS IS SPICY BUT NOT OVER-THE-TOP, eyes-watering kind of spicy. And when it's served with the bells and whistles that I suggest below, the heat calms down. This is great for the Stanley Cup playoffs, Super Bowl Sunday, or when you want to feed a crowd. If there are any leftovers, I make Stuffed Peppers (page 137) or freestyle a plate of nachos.

2 Tbsp canola oil

2 onions, diced

8 cloves garlic, diced

2 medium sweet potatoes, scrubbed and diced

1 Tbsp chipotle chili powder

1 Tbsp chili powder

1 tsp dried oregano leaves

1 tsp ground coriander

2 (28 fl oz/796 mL) cans San Marzano tomatoes

2 (19 fl oz/540 mL) cans no-salt-added black beans, rinsed and well drained

1 (10 fl oz/300 mL) jar whole roasted sweet peppers, diced, or 4 large roasted red peppers, diced

BELLS AND WHISTLES (PER SERVING)

¼ avocado, sliced

¼ cup fresh cilantro leaves, chopped

20 unsalted corn chips

¼ cup 0% plain Greek yogurt

1. Heat a 12- or 14-inch skillet over medium heat. Add the oil and onions and sauté until the onions start to soften, 3 to 5 minutes. Add the garlic and sweet potatoes and sauté until the sweet potatoes start to soften, 3 to 5 minutes. Add the chipotle chili powder, chili powder, oregano, and coriander. Sauté until the spices are well distributed. Transfer to a slow cooker, making sure to scrape up any of the browned bits on the bottom of the skillet.

2. Open the can of tomatoes and use a paring knife to roughly chop the tomatoes right in the can. Pour into the slow cooker.

3. Add the black beans and roasted red peppers, stir well, cover, and cook on low for 8 hours.

4. To serve, spoon the chili into deep bowls and top with any combination of the bells and whistles.

1 SERVING = 1 CUP WITHOUT THE BELLS AND WHISTLES
PER SERVING: 170 CALORIES, 3.3 G TOTAL FAT, 0.3 G SATURATED FAT, 0 G TRANS FAT, 0 MG CHOLESTEROL, 219 MG SODIUM, 29 G CARBOHYDRATE, 7.3 G FIBRE, 6.8 G SUGARS, 0 G ADDED SUGARS, 8 G PROTEIN, 736 MG POTASSIUM
CARBOHYDRATE CHOICE = 1½ CHOICES

1 SERVING = 1 CUP WITH THE BELLS AND WHISTLES
PER SERVING: 468 CALORIES, 19.1 G TOTAL FAT, 2.2 G SATURATED FAT, 0 G TRANS FAT, 0 MG CHOLESTEROL, 249 MG SODIUM, 58.8 G CARBOHYDRATE, 12.8 G FIBRE, 9.3 G SUGARS, 0 G ADDED SUGARS, 17 G PROTEIN, 1150 MG POTASSIUM
CARBOHYDRATE CHOICE = 3 CHOICES

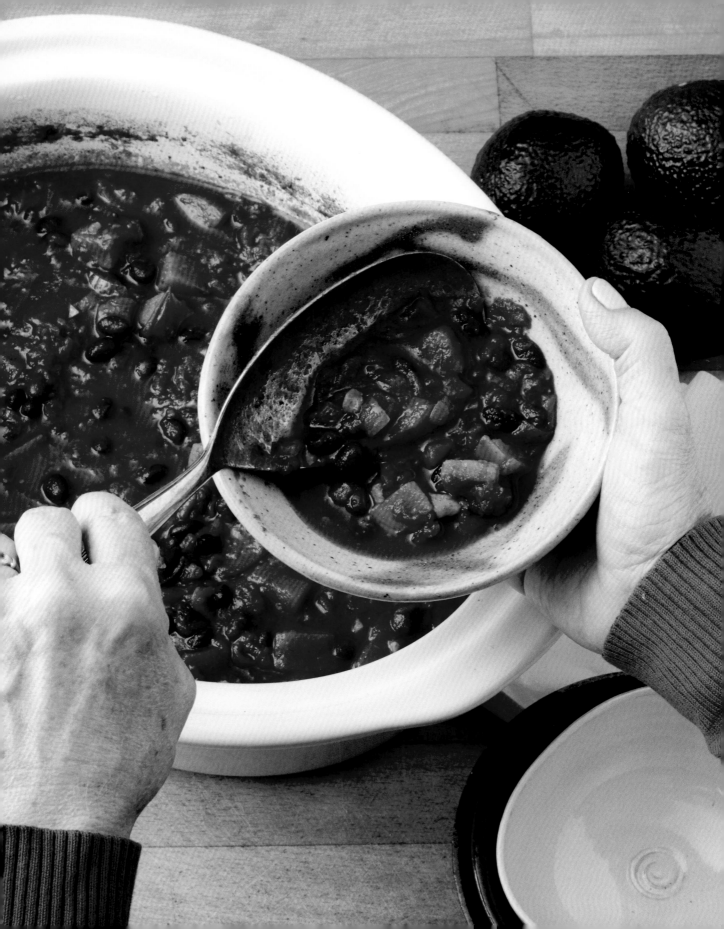

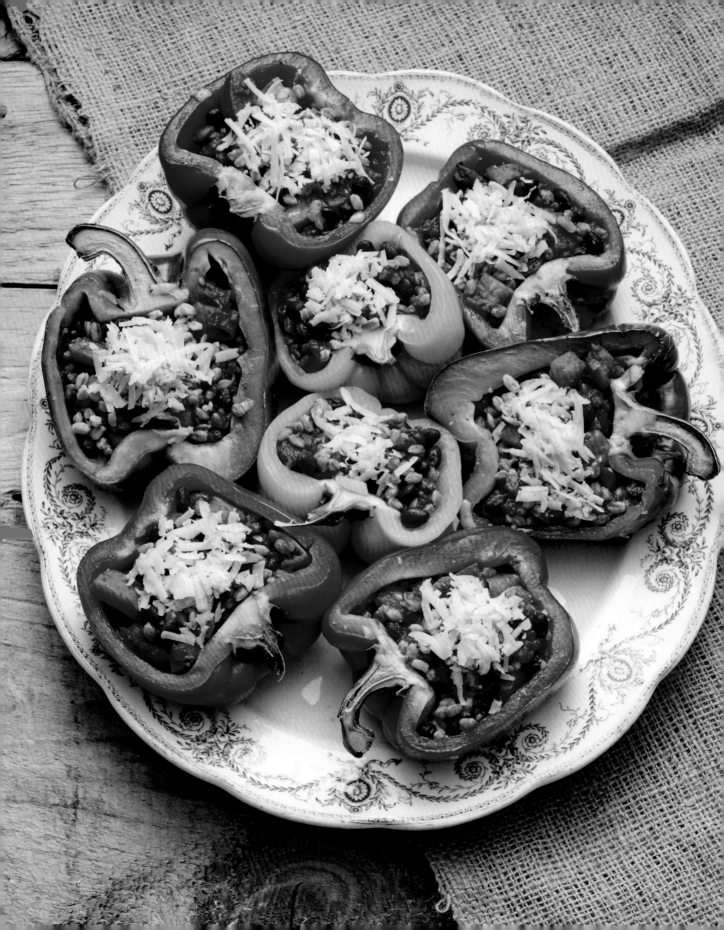

Stuffed Peppers   VEG · *Serves 4*

MOST NORTH AMERICAN FAMILIES THROW OUT 40% OF THEIR FOOD. Think about that. A whopping 40% of your food dollars plus the land, natural resources, time, and work that go into growing or raising that food to be delivered to a grocery store near you, only to be thrown out. To me, throwing food out is such a huge waste that I have created many recipes with repurposing them in mind. This recipe is a wonderful way to use leftover chili plus any leftover cooked grains you may have in the fridge.

4 large peppers

3 to 6 cups leftover Spicy Slow-Cooker Vegetarian Chili (page 134)

1 cup cooked whole grains (barley, wheat berries, farro, spelt) or quinoa (see page 13)

1 cup (4 oz/118 g) packed grated Monterey Jack cheese

NOTE: In September when the farmers' markets have local peppers, a large pepper can end up being humongous. I used the gargantuan peppers when we photographed this recipe and about 6 cups of leftover chili. Adjust the chili amount as needed to fit your peppers.

1. Preheat the oven to 350°F. Line a 9 × 13-inch casserole pan with wet parchment paper (see page 15).

2. Slice the peppers in half lengthwise through the stem. Remove and discard the seeds and membrane.

3. Boil 12 cups water in a large pot and cook the pepper halves for 5 minutes. Carefully drain and place into the prepared pan. Alternatively, you can place the peppers in a microwave-safe dish, cut sides down, with ¼ cup water and microwave on high for 5 to 8 minutes, until the peppers are slightly softened.

4. While the peppers are cooling down, combine the chili and the whole grains or quinoa in a large bowl.

5. Scoop out ½ cup of the mixture and place into each pepper half. Cover with a piece of wet parchment paper (see page 15) and bake for 35 minutes. Remove the parchment paper and sprinkle the peppers with cheese. Return to the oven and bake for about 10 minutes, until the cheese has melted. Serve immediately.

1 SERVING = 2 HALF PEPPERS
PER SERVING: 338 CALORIES, 12.1 G TOTAL FAT, 5.8 G SATURATED FAT, 0 G TRANS FAT, 26 MG CHOLESTEROL, 343 MG SODIUM, 43.3 G CARBOHYDRATE, 10.2 G FIBRE, 9.3 G SUGARS, 0 G ADDED SUGARS, 12.3 G PROTEIN, 1053 MG POTASSIUM
CARBOHYDRATE CHOICE = 2 CHOICES

Chicken & Chickpea Curry LF GF · *Serves 4*

MY MOM CALLED HERSELF A "PLAIN COOK." She thought pepper was an exotic spice. When I tasted Indian cuisine for the first time, it blew my mind. The flavour combinations rocked my taste-bud world and made me a fan for life.

SPICE BLEND

1 Tbsp ground coriander

2 tsp ground turmeric

2 tsp freshly ground black pepper

2 tsp ground cumin

¼ tsp red pepper flakes

¼ tsp table salt

CHICKEN CURRY

1 large sweet potato, well scrubbed

2 onions

3 Tbsp canola oil

8 oz (225 g) skinless, boneless chicken thighs, cut in 1-inch chunks

8 cloves garlic, minced

2 Tbsp grated fresh ginger

2 cups chopped Roma tomatoes (about 5 large)

1 (19 fl oz/540 mL) can no-salt-added chickpeas, rinsed and well drained

1 (13½ fl oz/400 mL) can low-fat coconut milk (shake well before opening)

1 cup frozen baby peas

2 cups cooked quinoa or barley, for serving (see page 13)

Hot sauce, for serving (optional)

1. Make the spice blend. Combine the coriander, turmeric, pepper, cumin, red pepper flakes, and salt in a small bowl. Set aside.

2. Cut the sweet potato in half, then into ½-inch pieces. You should get about 4 cups. Set aside. Cut the onions in half, then thinly slice each half into half moons.

3. Heat a large 12- or 14-inch skillet over medium-high heat. When the pan is hot, add the oil and chicken. Cook for 3 to 6 minutes, until the chicken is browned.

4. Reduce heat to medium, add the onions and garlic, and sauté until the onions turn golden brown, 3 to 6 minutes.

5. Add the ginger, sweet potatoes, and spice blend. Mix well. Add the tomatoes and sauté until they start to break down and release their juices, about 2 minutes.

6. Add the chickpeas and coconut milk, and make sure you scrape up any browned bits on the bottom of the skillet—they are loaded with flavour and if you scrape them up now, the dish will taste better and it won't burn on the bottom.

7. Bring the curry to a boil, cover, reduce heat to medium-low, and simmer for 20 minutes, stirring occasionally.

8. Remove the lid and simmer for an additional 15 minutes, adjusting the heat as needed.

9. Stir in the frozen peas, remove from heat, and let sit, covered, until the peas are heated through. Serve over cooked quinoa or barley. Add hot sauce if desired. Store any leftovers in the fridge for up to 3 days.

1 SERVING = ¼ OF THE RECIPE WITHOUT QUINOA OR BARLEY
PER SERVING: 487 CALORIES, 22.8 G TOTAL FAT, 6.7 G SATURATED FAT, 0 G TRANS FAT, 53 MG CHOLESTEROL, 326 MG SODIUM, 48.3 G CARBOHYDRATE, 10.3 G FIBRE, 9.6 G SUGARS, 0 G ADDED SUGARS, 23.3 G PROTEIN, 887 MG POTASSIUM
CARBOHYDRATE CHOICE = 2½ CHOICES

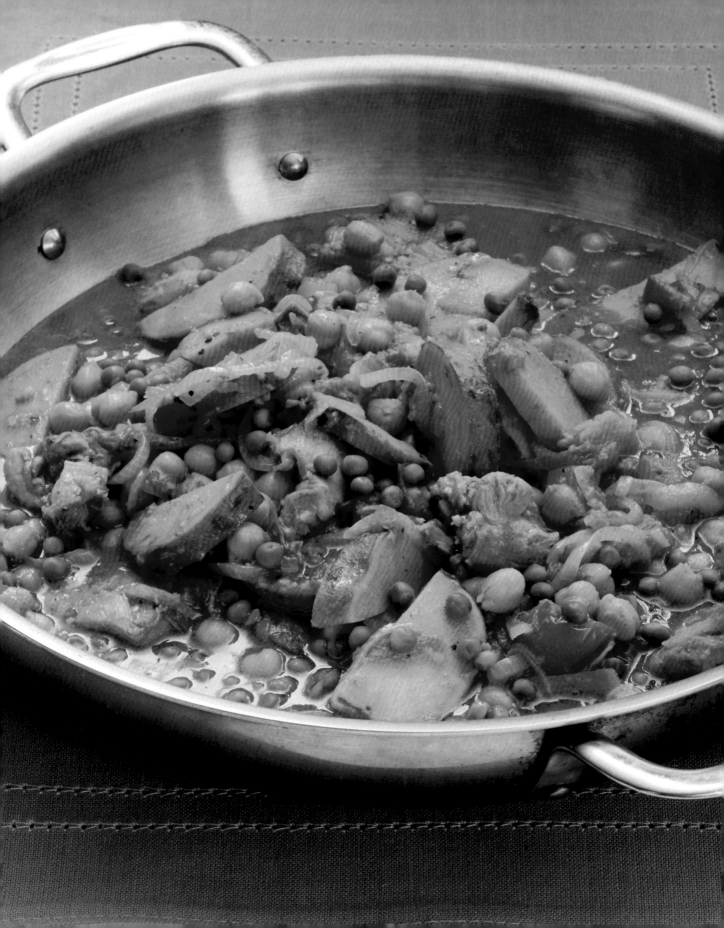

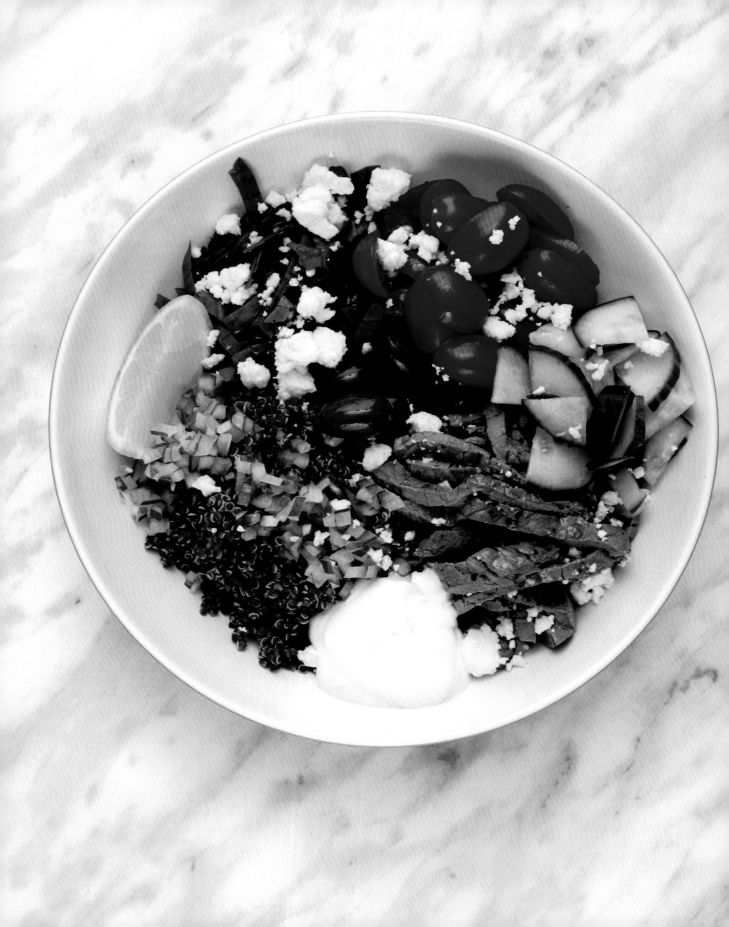

Mediterranean-Style Buddha Bowl *Serves 4*

THE BUDDHA BOWL CRAZE IS ONE OF MY FAVOURITE FOOD TRENDS. To me, it's a comfort meal all tucked into one pretty bowl. This recipe is the easiest and the most protein-dense of the four Buddha bowl recipes in the book; it's all about assembly. Use leftover cooked beef, cooked quinoa, and store-bought tzatziki. It's great for those nights when you're in a rush.

HAVE ON HAND FOR THE 4 BOWLS

2 cups cooked quinoa
(see page 13)

10 oz (283 g) leftover
cooked steak, thinly sliced

FOR THE 4 BOWLS

2 cups baby spinach, julienned

16 Kalamata olives, pitted

2 cups grape tomatoes, halved

½ cup diced red onion

¼ large English cucumber,
quartered and thinly sliced

½ cup (3 oz/85 g) crumbled feta
cheese

½ cup tzatziki

¼ cup extra virgin olive oil

½ large lemon, cut in 4 wedges

1. To assemble the bowls, you're going to equally divide all the ingredients. Each bowl should contain ½ cup quinoa, one-quarter of the sliced beef, one-quarter of the spinach, 4 olives, ½ cup tomatoes, 2 Tbsp red onion, and one-quarter of the cucumbers.

2. Sprinkle 2 Tbsp crumbled feta over top of each bowl, and spoon 2 Tbsp tzatziki on the side. Drizzle each bowl with 1 Tbsp olive oil and serve with a lemon wedge.

1 SERVING = 1 BOWL
PER SERVING: 528 CALORIES, 31.8 G TOTAL FAT, 10.2 G SATURATED FAT, 0 G TRANS FAT,
91 MG CHOLESTEROL, 629 MG SODIUM, 29 G CARBOHYDRATE, 4.4 G FIBRE, 5.6 G SUGARS,
0 G ADDED SUGARS, 31.3 G PROTEIN, 798 MG POTASSIUM
CARBOHYDRATE CHOICE = 1½ CHOICES

Middle Eastern–Style Buddha Bowl VEG LF · *Serves 4*

I CREATED THIS BUDDHA BOWL FOR THE CHICKPEA LOVERS in the crowd. The combination of roasted chickpeas and tahini sauce along with lemony cauliflower put this near and dear to my chickpea-loving heart.

HAVE ON HAND FOR THE 4 BOWLS

2 cups cooked quinoa
(see page 13)

4 cups Roasted Cauliflower with Lemon & Almonds (page 164)

½ cup diced red onion

1 cup coarsely chopped fresh parsley leaves

TAHINI SAUCE

¼ cup + 2 Tbsp tahini

¼ cup fresh lemon juice

1 tsp liquid honey

1 tsp Tabasco sauce

⅛ tsp table salt

CHICKPEAS

2 Tbsp canola oil

1 tsp ground turmeric

1 tsp ground coriander

1 tsp freshly ground black pepper

1 (19 fl oz/540 mL) can no-salt-added chickpeas, rinsed and well drained

1. Prepare the tahini sauce. Whisk together the tahini, lemon juice, ¼ cup water, honey, Tabasco, and salt. Set aside.

2. To prepare the chickpeas, heat a 12- or 14-inch non-stick skillet over medium heat. Add the oil, turmeric, coriander, and pepper and mix to combine. Add the chickpeas and sauté until the chickpeas are heated through and starting to get slightly crispy. It takes about 5 minutes and you will hear popping.

3. Remove the chickpeas from the heat and start assembling the four bowls. Each bowl should contain ½ cup quinoa, 1 cup roasted cauliflower, ½ cup chickpeas, and 2 Tbsp red onion. Sprinkle each with ¼ cup parsley and 3 heaping Tbsp tahini sauce.

1 SERVING = 1 BOWL
PER SERVING: 513 CALORIES, 27.6 G TOTAL FAT, 2.9 G SATURATED FAT, 0 G TRANS FAT, 0 MG CHOLESTEROL, 202 MG SODIUM, 53.6 G CARBOHYDRATE, 10.4 G FIBRE, 5 G SUGARS, 1.5 G ADDED SUGARS, 17.5 G PROTEIN, 695 MG POTASSIUM
CARBOHYDRATE CHOICE = 3 CHOICES

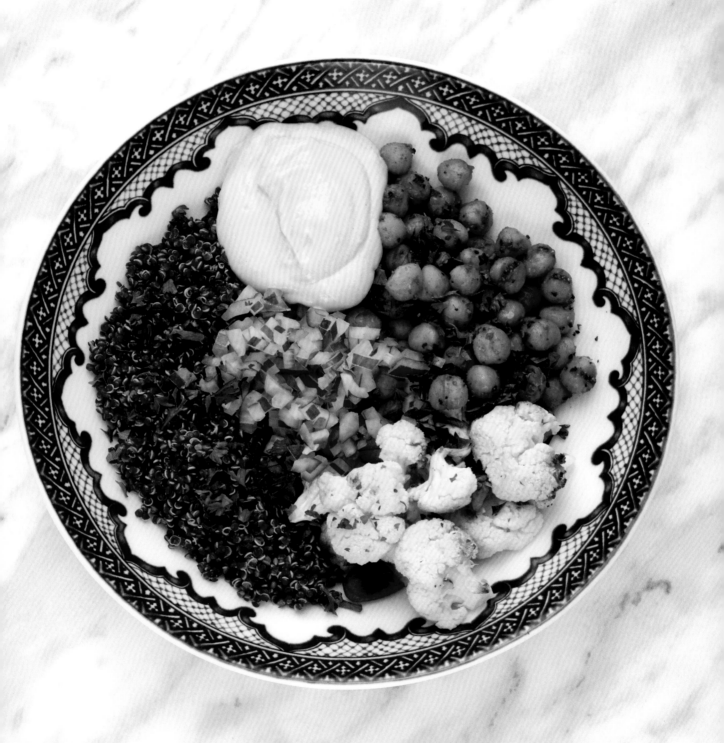

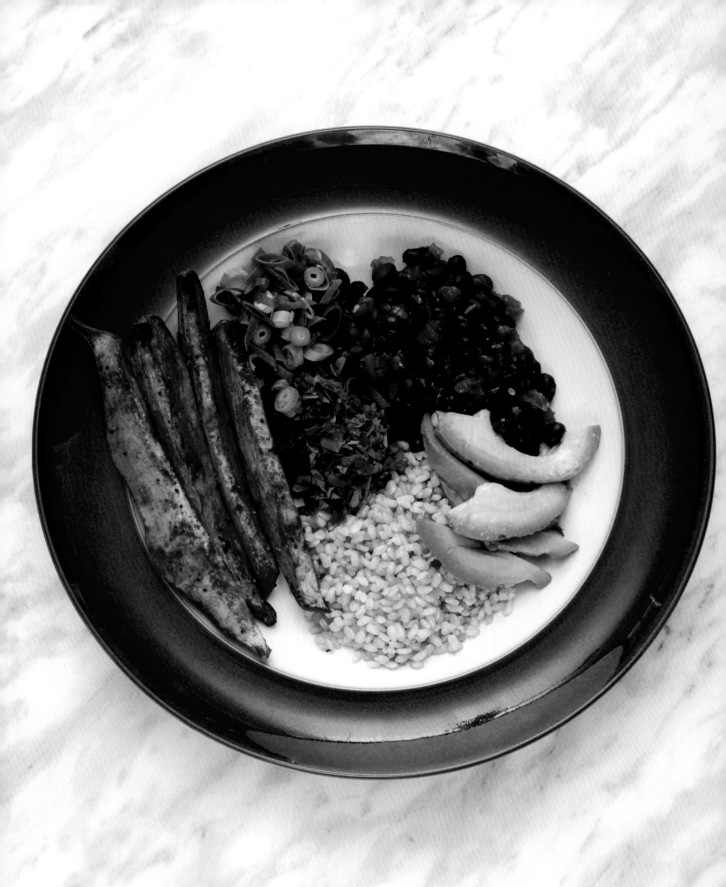

Mexican-Style Buddha Bowl VEG LF GF · *Serves 4*

WHENEVER AVOCADOS ARE IN SEASON, I immediately start craving this Buddha bowl. For fans of Mexican food, this one has your name on it. And if you prefer Mexican food that isn't too spicy, you're going to love this.

HAVE ON HAND FOR THE 4 BOWLS

4 sweet potatoes, quartered lengthwise and roasted

2 cups cooked brown rice (see page 13)

SALAD DRESSING

2 Tbsp fresh lime juice

2 Tbsp canola oil

1 tsp liquid honey

BLACK BEAN SALAD

1 (19 fl oz/540 mL) can no-salt-added black beans, rinsed and well drained

½ cup low-sodium salsa

1 cup fresh cilantro leaves, chopped

1 large avocado, thinly sliced

2 green onions, whites included, thinly sliced

1. Prepare or reheat the sweet potato wedges in a frying pan over medium heat.

2. Prepare the salad dressing. Whisk together the lime juice, oil, and honey. Set aside. This can be made up to 2 days in advance.

3. Reheat the rice in the microwave or use it cold from the fridge.

4. In a medium bowl, toss together the black beans and salsa.

5. Assemble the four bowls. Each bowl should contain ½ cup brown rice, four sweet potato wedges, one-quarter of the black bean mixture, ¼ cup cilantro, one-quarter of the avocado, and one-quarter of the green onions. Drizzle each bowl with 1 Tbsp salad dressing and serve.

1 SERVING = 1 BOWL
PER SERVING: 480 CALORIES, 19.3 G TOTAL FAT, 2 G SATURATED FAT, 0 G TRANS FAT,
0 MG CHOLESTEROL, 53 MG SODIUM, 65.2 G CARBOHYDRATE, 13.6 G FIBRE, 6 G SUGARS,
1.5 G ADDED SUGARS, 14 G PROTEIN, 1419 MG POTASSIUM
CARBOHYDRATE CHOICE = 3½ CHOICES

South Asian–Style Buddha Bowl VEG GF · *Serves 5*

THE MAIN INGREDIENT IN THIS BUDDHA BOWL IS DAL. One of the tricks for making a fabulous dal is to have all your ingredients ready and waiting to hit the skillet. Once you turn on the heat, this recipe can be ready in about 15 minutes. Unlike the other Buddha bowl dinners, this makes five servings. I love that the fifth serving can serve as lunch the next day.

HAVE ON HAND FOR THE 5 BOWLS

2½ cups cooked quinoa or red basmati rice (see page 13)

SPICE BLEND

1½ tsp dry mustard

1½ tsp ground turmeric

1½ tsp ground cumin

1 tsp freshly ground black pepper

1 tsp ground cinnamon

½ tsp ground coriander

1 tsp table salt

⅛ tsp red pepper flakes (optional)

CUCUMBER MINT SALAD

½ cup 0% plain Greek yogurt

2 Tbsp thinly sliced fresh mint leaves

½ English cucumber, thinly sliced

DAL

2 Tbsp canola oil

2 onions, diced

6 cloves garlic, minced

2 Tbsp well-packed grated fresh ginger

1 cup dried red lentils, rinsed and well drained

2 cups whole grape tomatoes

2 cups packed Swiss chard or spinach, rinsed, leaves removed, and thinly sliced (optional)

1. To make the spice blend, whisk together the dry mustard, turmeric, cumin, pepper, cinnamon, coriander, salt, and red pepper flakes if using. Set aside.

2. To make the cucumber mint salad, mix together the yogurt and mint in a medium bowl. Add the cucumber slices and stir until the cucumber slices are well coated with the yogurt. Store, covered, in the fridge.

3. To make the dal, heat a 12- or 14-inch non-stick skillet over medium heat. Add the oil and onions and sauté for 3 to 5 minutes, until the onions start to turn golden brown. Add the garlic, ginger, and spice blend. Stir well.

4. Add 2½ cups water, scraping up any browned bits from the bottom of the pan with a wooden spoon. This will help prevent the dal from sticking. Add the lentils and tomatoes and stir to combine. Bring to a boil, cover, reduce heat to low, and cook for 10 minutes. Remove the lid and, using the back of the wooden spoon, smash each tomato and stir well. Cover and cook for another 5 minutes. Remove from heat, add Swiss chard or spinach, if using, and stir until it has wilted.

5. Assemble the five bowls. Each bowl will contain ½ cup cooked quinoa or basmati rice, one-fifth of the dal, and one-fifth of the cucumber mint salad.

1 SERVING = 1 BOWL WITH RED BASMATI RICE
PER SERVING: 374 CALORIES, 7.8 G TOTAL FAT, 0.7 G SATURATED FAT, 0 G TRANS FAT, 0 MG CHOLESTEROL, 526 MG SODIUM, 59.7 G CARBOHYDRATE, 8.7 G FIBRE, 4.1 G SUGARS, 0 G ADDED SUGARS, 18.7 G PROTEIN, 656 MG POTASSIUM
CARBOHYDRATE CHOICE = 3½ CHOICES

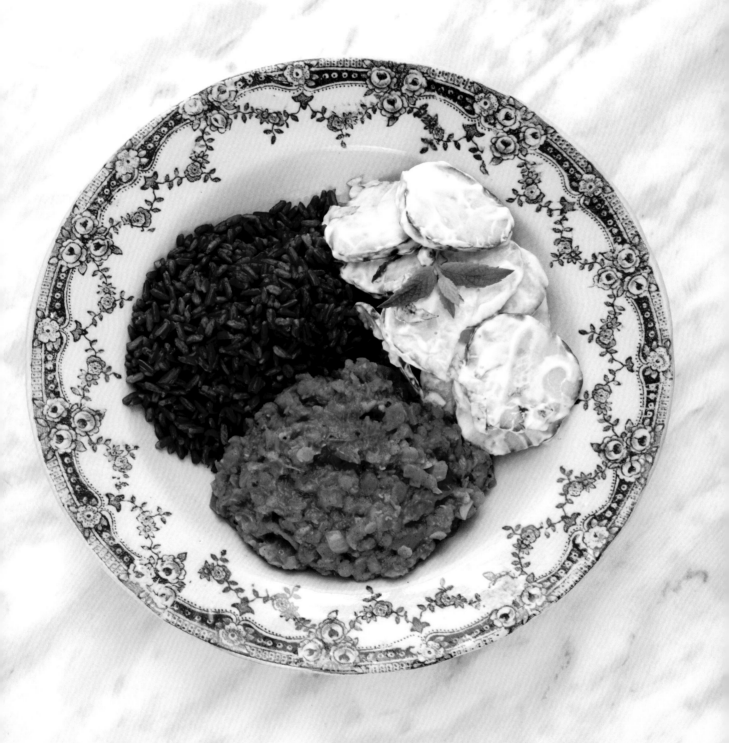

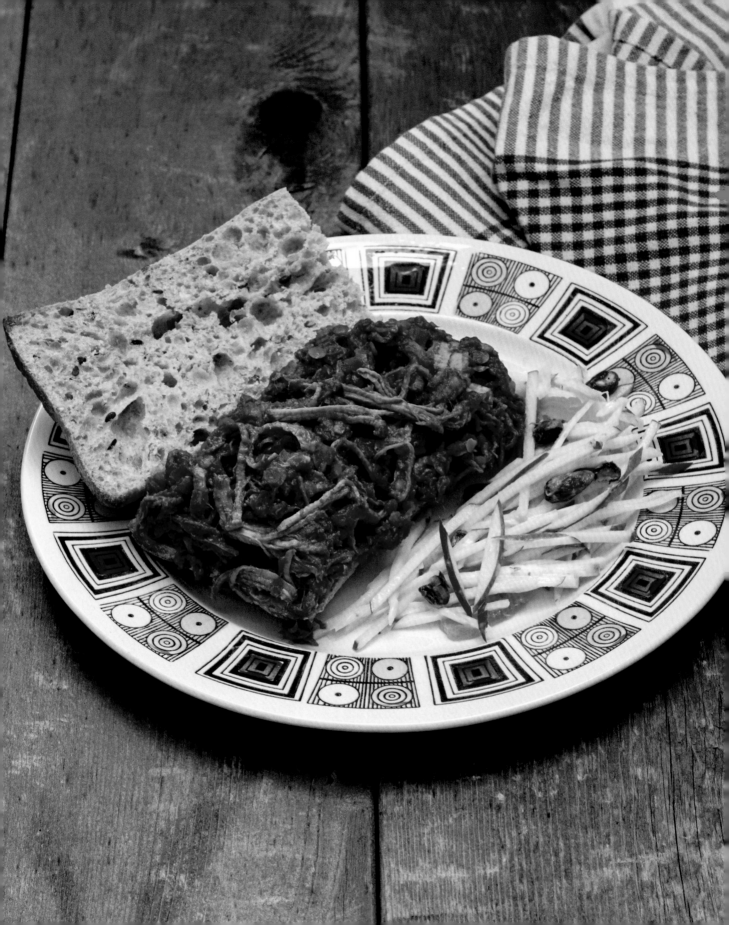

Slow-Cooker Pulled Pork   LF · *Serves 9*

FOR ALL YOU PULLED-PORK PUNDITS OUT THERE, this is my spin on the classic recipe. The cut of pork got a makeover from the usual pork shoulder to the leaner and more heart-healthy pork tenderloin, and because I'm me, I added red lentils to up the fibre. The lentils don't totally disappear, but they do add a smooth texture to the pork. Serve on a whole grain ciabatta bun with Springtime Apple & Fennel Slaw with Dried Apricots & Pistachios (page 107) on the side.

½ cup low-sodium ketchup

1 (28 fl oz/796 mL) can crushed tomatoes

1 Tbsp + 2 tsp smoked paprika

2 tsp dry mustard

1 tsp freshly ground black pepper

1 tsp chili powder

1 Tbsp Worcestershire sauce

1 Tbsp lower-sodium or lite tamari

2 Tbsp molasses

2 Tbsp pure amber maple syrup

2 Tbsp pure apple cider vinegar

1 cup dried red lentils, rinsed and well drained

1 onion, diced

2 cloves garlic, minced

2 lb (900 g) pork tenderloin

9 whole grain ciabatta buns, for serving (see sidebar)

✳

CAN'T FIND WHOLE GRAIN ciabatta buns? Use two ciabatta baguettes and cut them into nine equal pieces.

1. Pour the ketchup and tomatoes into a slow cooker and mix well. Add the paprika, dry mustard, pepper, and chili powder and stir well.

2. Add the Worcestershire, tamari, molasses, maple syrup, and apple cider vinegar and mix well. Stir in the lentils. Add the onion and garlic and, you guessed it, stir in.

3. Cut the pork tenderloin into four equal pieces on a separate cutting board. Then slice down the centre of each piece, but not through. Add the pork tenderloin to the slow cooker and make sure you submerge the pieces. Wash the cutting board and your hands, put the lid on the slow cooker, and set for 8 hours on low.

4. When the timer goes off, remove the pork and shred it using two forks. The pork will be almost falling apart. Add the pork back to the liquid in the slow cooker and stir in well. Cover and let sit for at least 15 minutes before serving on ciabatta buns. Freeze any leftover pulled pork for up to 3 months.

1 SERVING = 1 CUP ON A CIABATTA BUN
PER SERVING: 501 CALORIES, 5.4 G TOTAL FAT, 1.6 G SATURATED FAT, 0 G TRANS FAT, 63 MG CHOLESTEROL, 646 MG SODIUM, 70 G CARBOHYDRATE, 5.9 G FIBRE, 19.8 G SUGARS, 5.7 G ADDED SUGARS, 33.2 G PROTEIN, 1034 MG POTASSIUM
CARBOHYDRATE CHOICE = 4 CHOICES

Skillet Enchiladas   VEG · *Serves 6*

THIS RECIPE CALLS FOR LEFTOVER COOKED BARLEY, wheat berries, or quinoa to get this show on the road ASAP. If you aren't in a hurry, serve it with cornbread (page 74). Make the cornbread before you start the enchiladas; when the cornbread comes out of the oven, reduce the heat to 350°F and you are ready to go with the enchiladas. The cornbread cools as the cheese on the enchiladas melts—it's all about timing.

1½ cups fresh cooked or thawed frozen corn

1 Tbsp canola oil

1 small red onion, diced

6 cloves garlic, minced

1 large red pepper, diced

2 tsp chili powder

2 tsp ground cumin

2 tsp ground coriander

1 tsp freshly ground black pepper

1¼ cups canned enchilada sauce, mild, medium, or hot (see note)

1 (19 fl oz/540 mL) can no-salt-added black beans, rinsed and well drained

1 cup cooked pot barley, wheat berries, or quinoa (see page 13)

2 cups (8 oz/225 g) packed grated jalapeño Monterey Jack or Havarti cheese

1. Heat a 12- or 14-inch ovenproof skillet over medium heat. Add the corn and fry until it starts to blacken, 6 to 8 minutes.

2. Add the oil, red onion, and garlic and sauté until the onion begins to soften, 3 to 5 minutes.

3. Add the red pepper and continue sautéing until the red pepper starts to soften, 3 to 5 minutes. Add the chili powder, cumin, coriander, and pepper.

4. Pour in the enchilada sauce, black beans, and cooked barley (or whatever you decide to use) and stir in well. Cover with a lid, reduce heat to low, and simmer for 8 to 10 minutes or until heated through. Meanwhile, preheat the oven to 350°F.

5. Remove the lid and sprinkle with the cheese. Place in the oven, uncovered, to let the cheese melt, about 10 minutes. Remove from the oven, let sit for 5 minutes, and serve.

NOTE: You can find enchilada sauce in most large grocery stores or Latin American specialty grocery stores. Depending on the size of the can, freeze any leftover sauce.

1 SERVING = ⅙ OF THE RECIPE WITH COOKED BARLEY
PER SERVING: 357 CALORIES, 15.7 G TOTAL FAT, 3.7 G SATURATED FAT, 0 G TRANS FAT, 13 MG CHOLESTEROL, 675 MG SODIUM, 43 G CARBOHYDRATE, 9.5 G FIBRE, 3.5 G SUGARS, 0.9 G ADDED SUGARS, 15.7 G PROTEIN, 610 MG POTASSIUM
CARBOHYDRATE CHOICE = 2 CHOICES

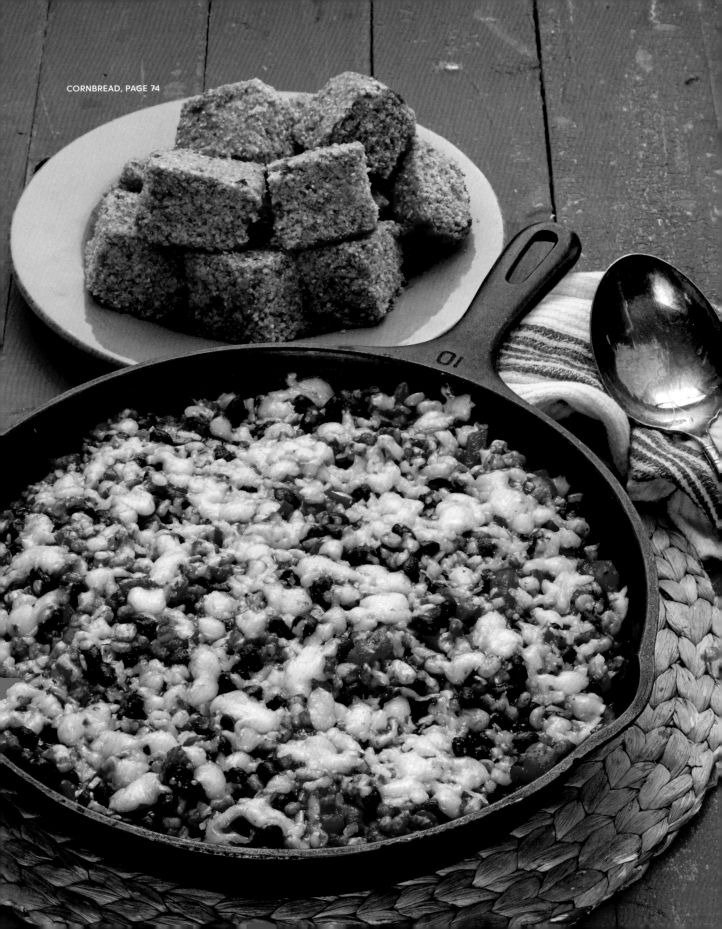

CORNBREAD, PAGE 74

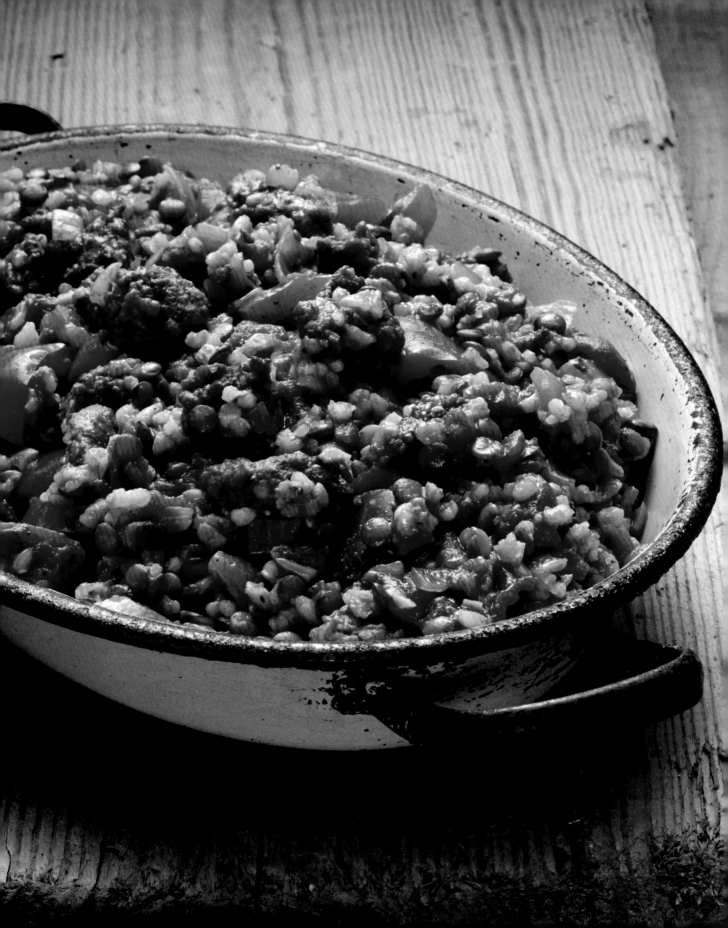

Chorizo, Brown Rice & Lentils LF · *Serves 6 or 7*

I'M A FAN OF ONE-POT DINNERS. Chop, sauté, cover, and walk away while the stove does the cooking for you. Sit down with a good book, have a cocktail with your significant other, or just lollygag about for 45 to 50 minutes, and the next thing you know you are serving a full-course dinner.

SPICE MIXTURE

2 tsp ground cumin

1 tsp ground coriander

1 tsp ancho chili powder

½ tsp dried basil leaves

½ tsp dried oregano leaves

¼ tsp smoked paprika

¼ tsp table salt

¼ tsp freshly ground black pepper

13 oz (370 g) chorizo sausage, mild, medium, or spicy (about 2 sausages)

1 large onion, chopped

4 large cloves garlic, minced

1 red pepper, chopped in 1½-inch pieces

1 green pepper, chopped in 1½-inch pieces

1 stalk celery, chopped

¾ cup short-grain brown rice, rinsed well and drained

1 cup dried green lentils, rinsed and well drained

1 (28 fl oz/796 mL) can no-salt-added diced tomatoes

1½ cups no-salt-added chicken or vegetable broth

1. Make the spice mixture. In a small bowl, whisk together the cumin, coriander, chili powder, basil, oregano, paprika, salt, and pepper.

2. On a separate cutting board and using a sharp knife, cut the casing of each sausage lengthwise, being careful not to cut all the way through. Heat a 12- or 14-inch deep-sided skillet over medium heat. Peel off the casings and drop the sausage meat into the hot skillet. Discard the casings and package and wash the cutting board and your hands.

3. Gently fry the sausage meat, breaking it up into pieces with a wooden spoon until browned and cooked through.

4. Add the onion, garlic, red and green peppers, and celery. Sauté until the onion is soft, 3 to 5 minutes. Add the spice mixture and stir to coat the vegetables. Sauté for 1 minute.

5. Add the rice, lentils, tomatoes, and broth. Stir well, making sure to scrape up any browned bits from the bottom of the pan—this will prevent it from burning as well as give the dish more flavour.

6. Bring to a boil, cover, and reduce heat to low. Cook for 40 to 45 minutes, until the liquid has been absorbed and the rice and lentils are tender but not mushy. Remove from heat, stir, cover, and let sit for 5 minutes. Store any leftovers in a covered container in the fridge for up to 3 days.

1 SERVING = 1½ CUPS
PER SERVING: 331 CALORIES, 6.4 G TOTAL FAT, 2.1 G SATURATED FAT, 0 G TRANS FAT, 20 MG CHOLESTEROL, 293 MG SODIUM, 53 G CARBOHYDRATE, 6.3 G FIBRE, 4.2 G SUGARS, 0 G ADDED SUGARS, 17.1 G PROTEIN, 792 MG POTASSIUM
CARBOHYDRATE CHOICE = 3 CHOICES

Festive Balls LF GF · *Serves 6*

EVERYONE LOVES MY FESTIVE BALLS. They smell amazing, have a great shape, and yes, I'm totally stealing this schtick from the iconic 1999 *Saturday Night Live* sketch. If you love turkey dinner with all the trimmings, serve these balls with Baked Sweet Potatoes with Apples & Cranberries (page 169) and Stir-Fried Brussels Sprouts with Bacon & Cranberries (page 174). Use your good dishes and get that celebratory feeling.

¾ cup finely diced cremini mushrooms

½ cup fresh or slightly thawed frozen cranberries, coarsely chopped

¼ cup finely diced celery

¼ cup flaxseed meal (see page 184)

2 Tbsp poultry seasoning

1 Tbsp canola oil

2 Tbsp pure amber maple syrup

1 onion, grated

½ tsp table salt

1 to 2 tsp freshly ground black pepper

1 lb (450 g) extra-lean ground turkey

1. Place a rack in the middle of the oven and preheat the oven to 350°F. Line a large rimmed baking sheet with parchment paper and set aside.

2. In a large bowl, mix together the mushrooms, cranberries, celery, flaxseed meal, poultry seasoning, oil, maple syrup, grated onion, salt, and pepper. Add the turkey and mix well.

3. Using a ¼-cup measure, scoop out 18 equally sized balls and place them onto the prepared baking sheet. I use a ¼-cup ice-cream scoop with a release button to make sure they are all the same size.

4. Bake for about 35 minutes or until a meat thermometer inserted into the middle of a meatball registers 172°F (which is higher than the recommended temperature, but it helps to firm up the meatball). Serve immediately. Any leftovers can be stored in the fridge for up to 3 days.

1 SERVING = 3 BALLS
PER SERVING: 206 CALORIES, 10.5 G TOTAL FAT, 2.2 G SATURATED FAT, 0 G TRANS FAT, 73 MG CHOLESTEROL, 223 MG SODIUM, 10.8 G CARBOHYDRATE, 2.9 G FIBRE, 5.6 G SUGARS, 4 G ADDED SUGARS, 16.9 G PROTEIN, 377 MG POTASSIUM
CARBOHYDRATE CHOICE = ½ CHOICE

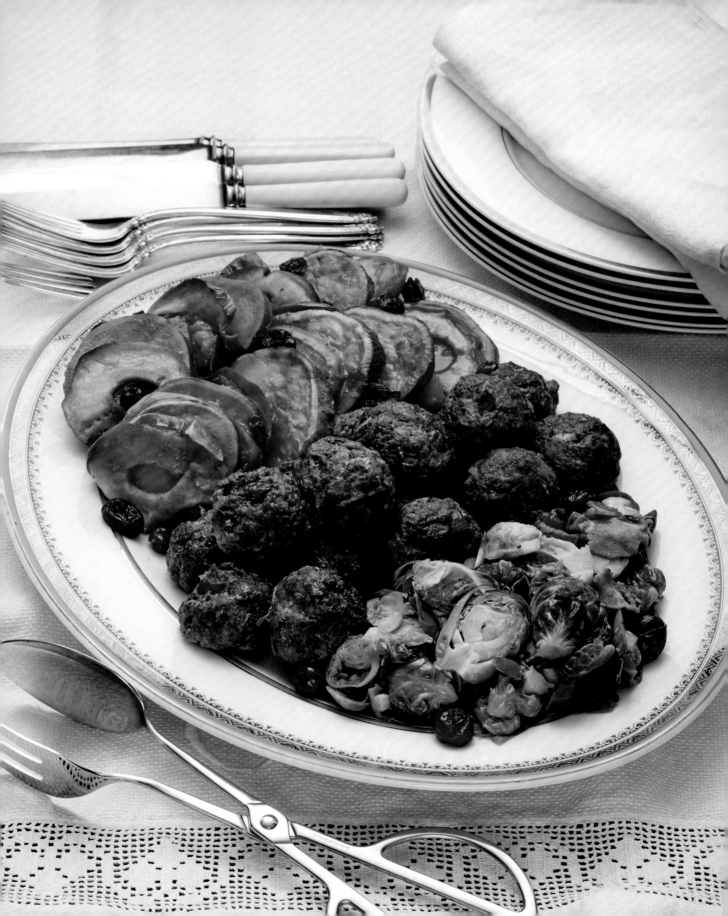

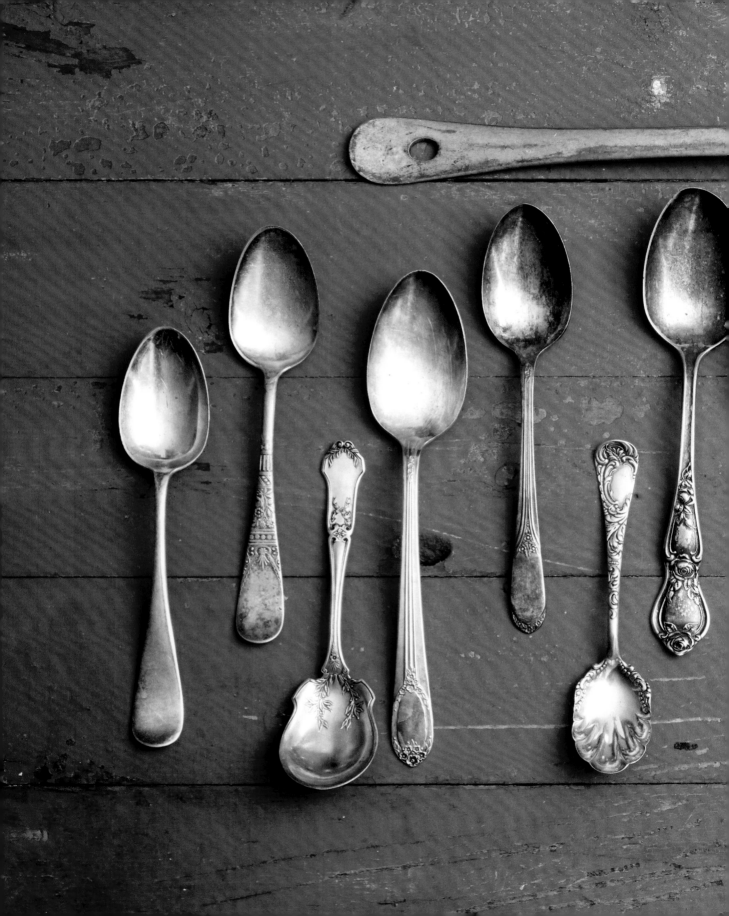

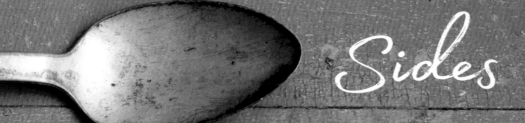

Sides

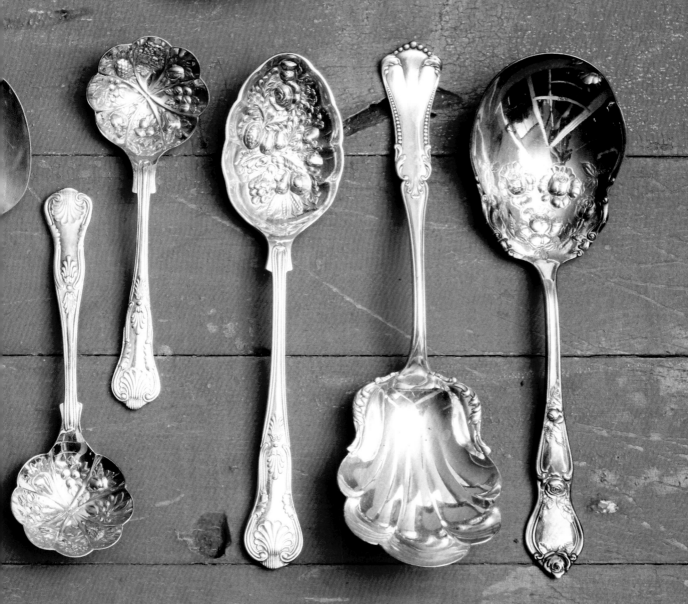

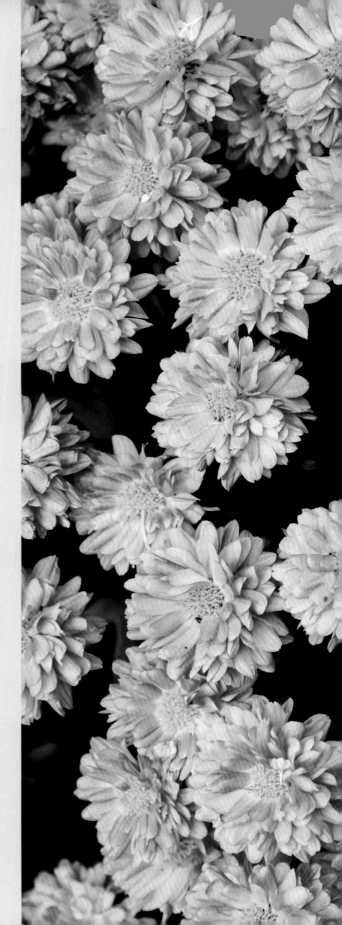

Did your mom ever yell at you to clean your plate and make sure you ate your cauliflower? My mom didn't have to yell at me—well, at least not about eating my cauliflower—because I liked my vegetables. I know, I know, I was a weird kid.

We know that eating vegetables and fruit can lower your chances of developing certain diseases like heart disease and cancer. We also know that eating an array of vegetables and fruit provides your body with vitamins and minerals, dietary fibre, and a veritable army of healthful substances, including plant sterols, flavonoids, and other antioxidants. So why aren't we running full steam to our nearest produce department to stock up?

One of the deterrents to eating more produce is the preparation time. Consumers want convenience. Luckily, this chapter is bursting with easy-to-make recipes that help you add those much-needed daily servings of vegetables and fruits to your dinner plate.

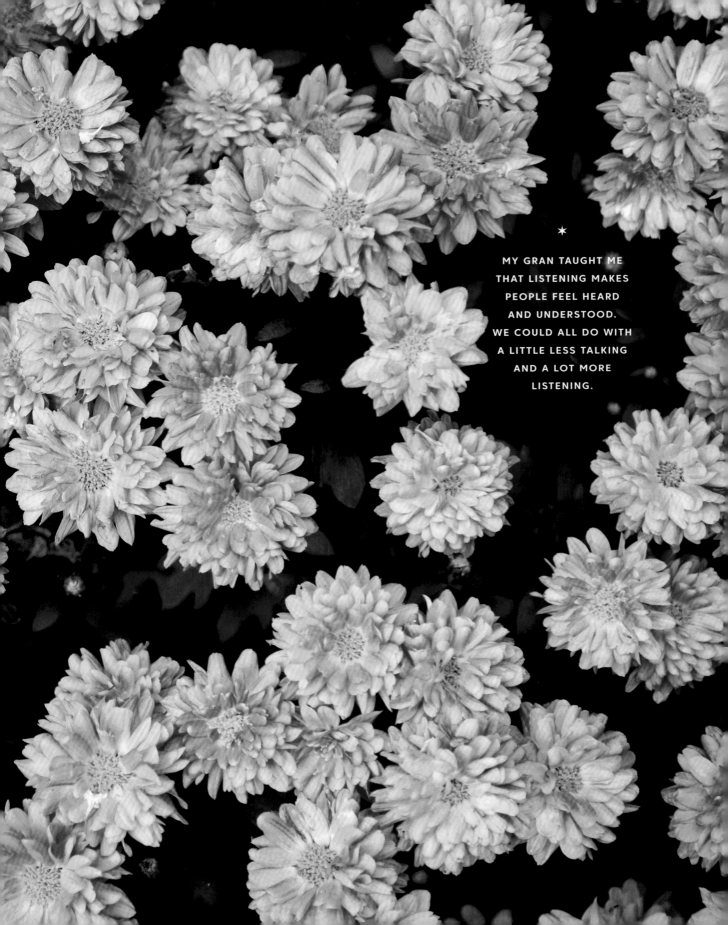

MY GRAN TAUGHT ME
THAT LISTENING MAKES
PEOPLE FEEL HEARD
AND UNDERSTOOD.
WE COULD ALL DO WITH
A LITTLE LESS TALKING
AND A LOT MORE
LISTENING.

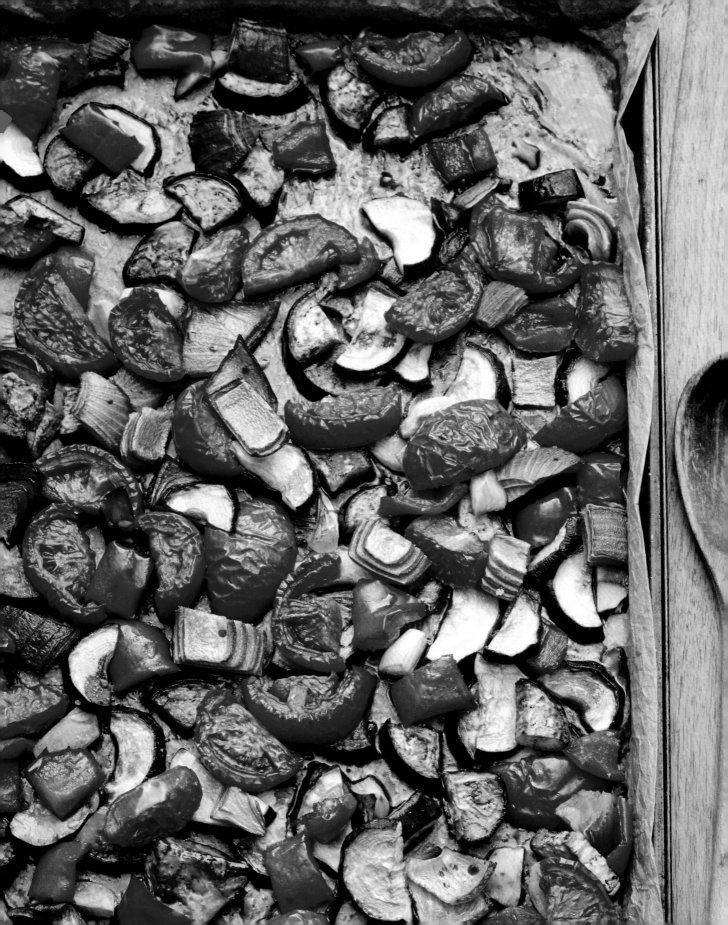

Ratatouille   VEG V LF GF · *Serves 8*

RATATOUILLE IS LIKE HAVING ALL THE FLAVOURS OF SUMMER IN ONE PAN. This iconic French dish is often cooked on the stovetop, but I love how the kitchen smells when you roast all these yummy vegetables. It's a caramelized yum fest.

1 small eggplant, rinsed, quartered, and cut in ½-inch slices

1 small zucchini, halved lengthwise and cut in ½-inch half moons

7 cloves garlic, halved

1 large red pepper, cut in 1-inch pieces

½ medium red onion, cut in 1-inch pieces

1 lb (450 g) Roma tomatoes, halved lengthwise and cut in 1-inch pieces

3 Tbsp extra virgin olive oil

3 Tbsp balsamic vinegar

1. Place a rack in the middle of your oven and preheat the oven to 325°F.

2. Line a rimmed baking sheet with wet parchment paper (see page 15).

3. Place the eggplant, zucchini, garlic, pepper, red onion, and tomatoes on the baking sheet. Drizzle with the oil and vinegar and toss to combine.

4. Bake in the preheated oven for 1½ hours, until the vegetables are very tender. No flipping required—this recipe is easy-peasy.

5. Serve hot or at room temperature. Any leftovers can be stored in the fridge for up to 3 days.

NOTE: In the summer, you can make this on the barbecue to avoid adding more heat to your kitchen. Just place the baking sheet with the vegetables over indirect heat (a burner that isn't on), close the lid, and roast as you would in the oven.

1 SERVING = ½ CUP
PER SERVING: 85 CALORIES, 5.5 G TOTAL FAT, 0 G SATURATED FAT, 0 G TRANS FAT,
0 MG CHOLESTEROL, 7 MG SODIUM, 9 G CARBOHYDRATE, 2.7 G FIBRE, 4.4 G SUGARS,
0 G ADDED SUGARS, 1.5 G PROTEIN, 361 MG POTASSIUM
CARBOHYDRATE CHOICE = ½ CHOICE

Zucchini Sticks VEG · *Serves 4*

MENTION WHITE SPOT IN A CONVERSATION and you'll quickly find out who's from Vancouver. The conversation will immediately include words like Zoo Sticks, Monty Mushroom Burgers, Chicken Pickens, or a side of pickles with extra Triple "O" sauce. White Spot, an iconic family restaurant that's been around since 1928, features in some of my favourite childhood memories. The car hop would slide long trays through the windows and you could eat right there in your car while the windows fogged up. Zoo Sticks, a White Spot classic, are deep-fried zucchini sticks served with a dill sauce. Here's my non-deep-fried spin on this classic.

4 medium zucchini

⅔ cup whole wheat panko crumbs

¼ cup flaxseed meal (see page 184)

¼ cup finely grated Parmigiano-Reggiano

½ tsp freshly ground black pepper

½ tsp garlic powder

½ tsp onion powder

3 Tbsp canola oil

DIPPING SAUCE

¼ cup 0% plain yogurt

¼ cup low-fat mayo

2 Tbsp finely chopped fresh dill

1. Place a rack in the middle of your oven and preheat the oven to 425°F. Line a rimmed baking sheet with parchment paper. Set aside.

2. Rinse and pat dry the zucchini. Remove the ends, cut each zucchini in half lengthwise, then cut each half into four wedges. You'll have 32 wedges in total.

3. In a shallow bowl or dish, mix together the panko crumbs, flaxseed meal, cheese, pepper, garlic powder, and onion powder.

4. Measure out the oil and place it in a small bowl.

5. Dip a pastry brush into the oil and then brush onto the cut sides of the zucchini (not the green peel). Press the zucchini firmly into the panko mixture, making sure that both cut sides are heavily covered with the crumbs. Place the zucchini wedges, peel side down, onto the prepared sheet and bake for 15 minutes.

6. While the zucchini sticks are in the oven, make the dipping sauce. Whisk together the yogurt, mayo, and dill.

7. When the zucchini sticks are ready, serve right away with the sauce. They're great as a side to burgers or as a snack while you are watching the Canucks. Okay, my Vancouver roots are really showing now.

1 SERVING = 8 PIECES WITH 1 TBSP DIPPING SAUCE
PER SERVING: 113 CALORIES, 6.4 G TOTAL FAT, 2.3 G SATURATED FAT, 0 G TRANS FAT, 14 MG CHOLESTEROL, 148 MG SODIUM, 8.1 G CARBOHYDRATE, 3 G FIBRE, 3.3 G SUGARS, 0.3 G ADDED SUGARS, 7 G PROTEIN, 351 MG POTASSIUM
CARBOHYDRATE CHOICE = < 1 CHOICE

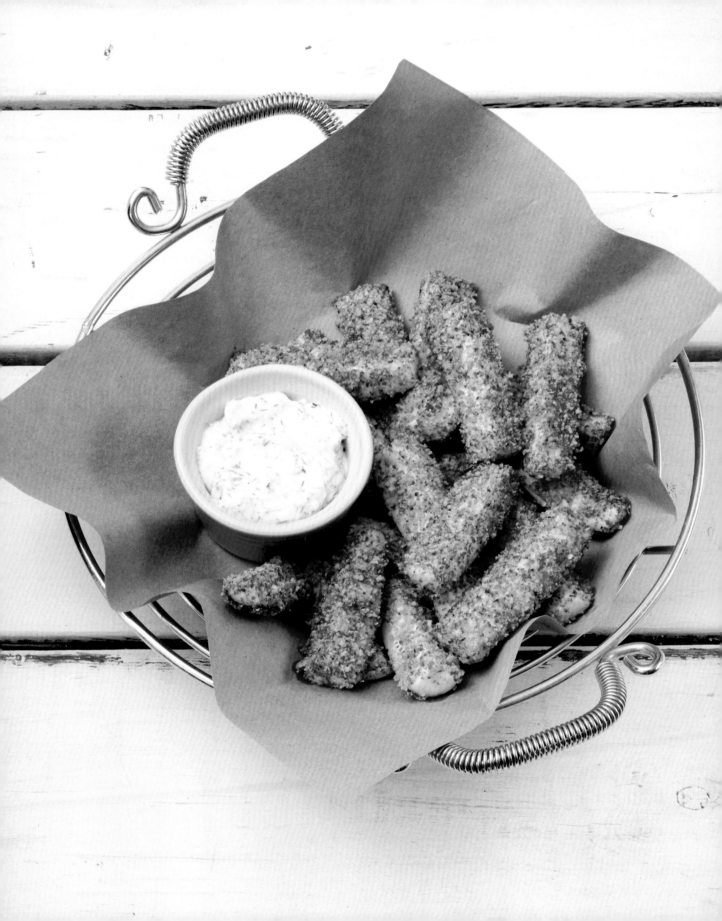

Roasted Cauliflower with Lemon & Almonds VEG V LF GF · *Serves 10*

I WAS INSPIRED TO CREATE THIS RECIPE AFTER THE ELEVENTH TIME I had been to Patria, a Spanish tapas restaurant in Toronto. They have this amazing dish that uses lemon and almonds. I kept ordering it until I came up with this alternative. I still drop by occasionally on a Friday night with my girlfriends for a glass of fabulous red wine and more tapas, but now it's a mission of fun, not food espionage.

1 large head cauliflower
2 Tbsp canola oil
¼ cup fresh lemon juice, divided
½ cup chopped raw almonds
1 Tbsp lemon zest

1. Place a rack in the middle of the oven and preheat the oven to 425°F. Line a rimmed baking sheet with wet parchment paper (see page 15).

2. Remove the outer leaves from the cauliflower. Cut it in half and remove the stalk. Cut the cauliflower into florets the size of a large walnut shell. Reserve the stalks for crudité or soup stock. You should have approximately 11 cups of florets (they will shrink as they cook).

3. Place the florets in a large bowl and toss with the oil.

4. Transfer the florets to the prepared baking sheet and drizzle with 3 Tbsp of the lemon juice. Sprinkle with the almonds. Bake for 20 minutes, remove from the oven, and gently flip the cauliflower. Drizzle with the remaining lemon juice.

5. Return the cauliflower to the oven and bake for an additional 10 minutes or until the florets are starting to turn brown and are soft. Remove from the oven, and sprinkle with the zest. Serve the entire cauliflower, or reserve 4 cups for the Middle Eastern-Style Buddha Bowl (page 142).

ONE SERVING = ½ CUP
PER SERVING: 68 CALORIES, 4.7 G TOTAL FAT, 0.3 G SATURATED FAT, 0 G TRANS FAT, 0 MG CHOLESTEROL, 18 MG SODIUM, 4.4 G CARBOHYDRATE, 1.7 G FIBRE, 1.4 G SUGARS, 0 G ADDED SUGARS, 2.3 G PROTEIN, 222 MG POTASSIUM
CARBOHYDRATE CHOICE = < 1 CHOICE

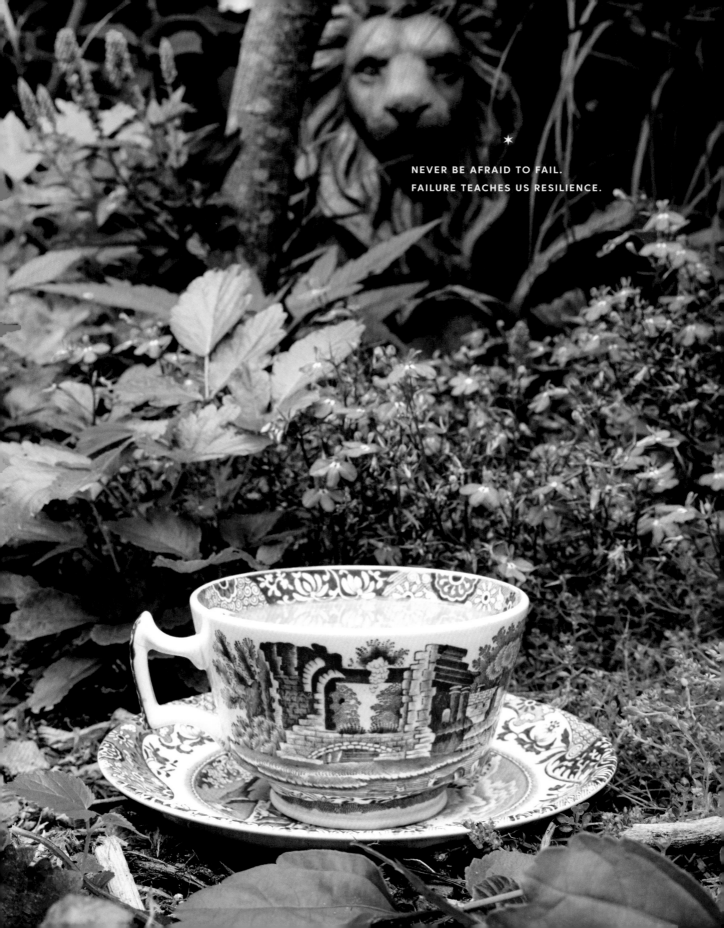

NEVER BE AFRAID TO FAIL.
FAILURE TEACHES US RESILIENCE.

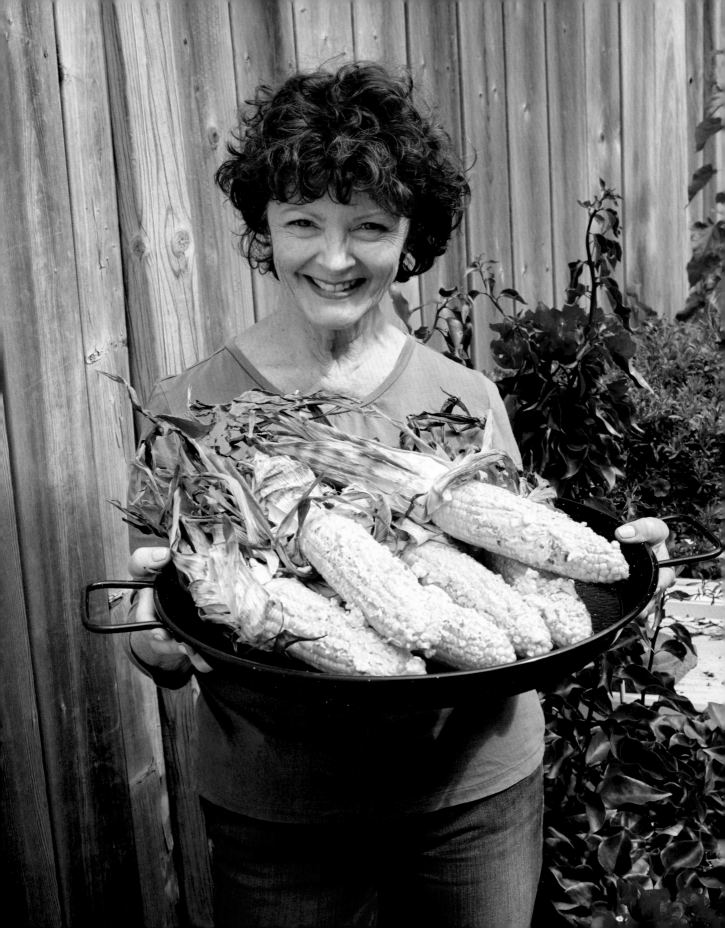

Mexican Street-Style Grilled Corn   VEG GF · *Serves 5*

MY HUSBAND AND I ARE ALWAYS ON THE LOOKOUT for new Mexican restaurants in Toronto. The first time we had Mexican street-style grilled corn was at a cute little place on College Street. We both took a bite, looked at each other, and said, "Oh, we've gotta make this at home." If you love Mexican food and grilled corn, this is a game changer.

5 large cobs fresh seasonal corn

CHIPOTLE CHEESE SAUCE
3 Tbsp 0% plain Greek yogurt
2 Tbsp low-fat mayo
1 Tbsp fresh lime juice
¾ tsp chipotle chili powder
½ cup (3 oz/85 g) well-packed crumbled feta, Manouri, or Cotija cheese

1. Preheat the barbecue to high.

2. Husk the corn. I like to leave part of the husk and stem on because it looks fabulous, but it's messy eating unless you are serving it outside.

3. Place the corn on the grill and reduce the heat to medium or 350°F. Close the lid and grill on all sides until the kernels start to char and the corn is getting soft, 8 to 12 minutes, depending on how big the kernels are.

4. While the corn is grilling, make the chipotle cheese sauce. In a medium bowl, mix together the yogurt, mayo, lime juice, chili powder, and cheese. I use an immersion blender to make sure the cheese is well distributed, but blending it with a wooden spoon works well too.

5. When the corn is ready, evenly spread about 2 Tbsp sauce onto each cob using a small spatula or knife. Serve right away with loads of napkins. This is messy to eat, but worth every moment.

1 SERVING = 1 COB
PER SERVING: 297 CALORIES, 7.8 G TOTAL FAT, 3 G SATURATED FAT, 0 G TRANS FAT, 16 MG CHOLESTEROL, 213 MG SODIUM, 53.4 G CARBOHYDRATE, 6.4 G FIBRE, 19.2 G SUGARS, 0.3 G ADDED SUGARS, 11 G PROTEIN, 618 MG POTASSIUM
CARBOHYDRATE CHOICE = 3 CHOICES

Oven-Roasted Butternut Squash VEG V LF GF · *Serves 10*

THIS SIDE-DISH RECIPE MAKES ENOUGH ROASTED SQUASH for dinner tonight AND the leftovers can be used in the Roasted Squash & Kale Salad with Pistachios & Fig Goat Cheese (page 123).

1 (4 lb/1.8 kg) butternut squash
2 Tbsp canola oil

SPICE MIX

1 tsp ground turmeric
½ tsp ground cinnamon
½ tsp freshly ground black pepper

1. Place a rack in the middle of the oven and preheat the oven to 425°F. Line a 9 × 13-inch rimmed baking sheet with wet parchment paper (see page 15) and set aside.

2. Rinse the squash under cold water and pat dry. Cut the long neck of the squash away from the bottom round part. Reserve the bottom part of the squash and roast it separately another day.

3. Using a sharp knife or a large peeler, cut off the thick peel. Cut the squash into 1-inch cubes. Place in a large bowl and add the oil. Toss to coat.

4. In a small bowl, combine the turmeric, cinnamon, and pepper. Sprinkle over the squash and transfer the squash to the baking sheet.

5. Roast for 25 to 30 minutes, until golden, and serve immediately. Leftovers will keep, covered, in the fridge for up to 3 days.

1 SERVING = ½ CUP
PER SERVING: 98 CALORIES, 3 G TOTAL FAT, 2 G SATURATED FAT, 0 G TRANS FAT,
0 MG CHOLESTEROL, 7 MG SODIUM, 19.3 G CARBOHYDRATE, 3.2 G FIBRE, 3.6 G SUGARS,
0 G ADDED SUGARS, 1.7 G PROTEIN, 521 MG POTASSIUM
CARBOHYDRATE CHOICE = 1 CHOICE

Baked Sweet Potatoes with Apples & Cranberries

VEG LF GF · *Serves 12*

SWEET POTATOES AND APPLES ARE A VEGETABLE AND FRUIT MARRIAGE MADE IN HEAVEN, especially around Thanksgiving. I've made a combo side dish using them for years, but it wasn't until my BFF Michale made a layered sweet potato and apple side dish that I decided to change up my recipe. So, with a big nod and a thank you to Michale, who has recipe-tested and helped me immensely throughout our 30-plus-year friendship in way more areas than food, here's my latest version of sweet potato and apples. See a picture on page 154.

3 medium sweet potatoes (about 2½ lb/1.1 kg)

6 Paula Red or McIntosh apples

1½ cups fresh or frozen cranberries

½ cup dried cranberries

¼ cup orange juice

2 Tbsp pure amber maple syrup

1. Place a rack in the middle of your oven and preheat the oven to 425°F. Line a 9 × 13-inch high-sided casserole dish with wet parchment paper (see page 15).

2. Scrub the sweet potatoes under cold running water, then cut into ½-inch slices. Set aside.

3. Rinse the apples well, pat dry, and core them using an apple corer. No apple corer? Do your best to remove only the core using a paring knife. Cut the apples into ½-inch slices.

4. You are going to make three rows of apple and sweet potato slices, leaning up against each other. Start with a slice of sweet potato and then place an apple slice against it. Continue until the entire pan is arranged in three lines.

5. Sprinkle fresh or frozen cranberries over top, tucking them in between the apples and sweet potatoes. Repeat with the dried cranberries.

6. Drizzle the orange juice and maple syrup over top.

7. Bake for 30 minutes, then remove from the oven and cover with a piece of wet parchment paper (see page 15). Return to the oven and bake for 25 to 30 minutes, until the sweet potatoes are tender. Let sit for 10 minutes before serving. Store any leftovers in the fridge for up to 3 days.

1 SERVING = ½ CUP
PER SERVING: 118 CALORIES, 0.2 G TOTAL FAT, 0 G SATURATED FAT, 0 G TRANS FAT, 0 MG CHOLESTEROL, 46 MG SODIUM, 29 G CARBOHYDRATE, 4.2 G FIBRE, 18.2 G SUGARS, 0.9 G ADDED SUGARS, 0.9 G PROTEIN, 247 MG POTASSIUM
CARBOHYDRATE CHOICE = 1½ CHOICES

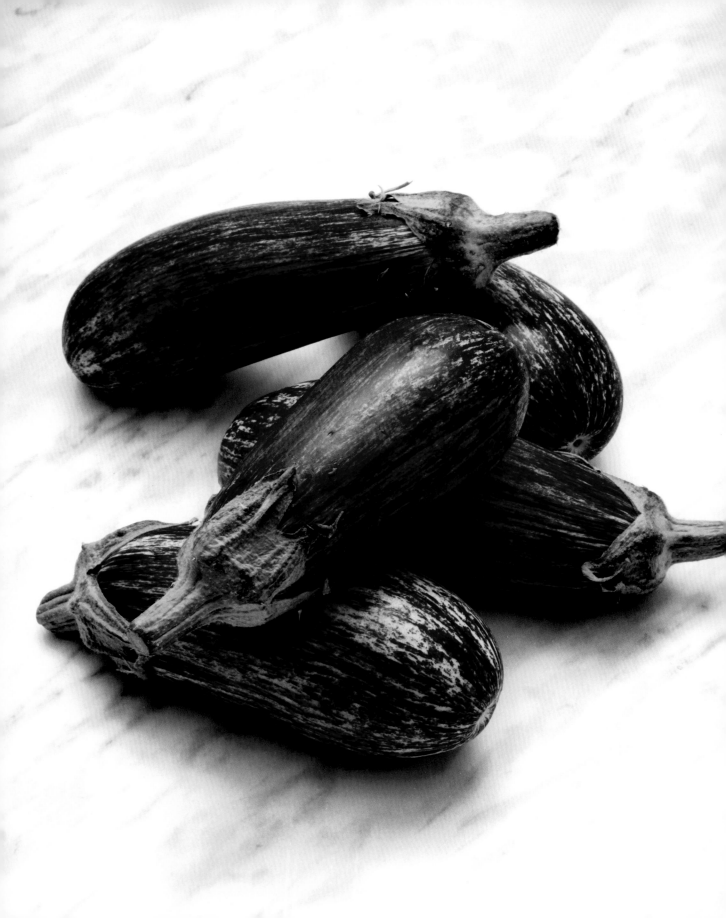

Eggplant Roll-Ups VEG GF • *Serves 6*

I USED TO THINK THAT EGGPLANT WAS A BORING VEGETABLE. It either didn't have much flavour, or it was bitter. To add insult to injury, there was all that salt you had to add to leach out the bitterness. Seriously, too much work for a vegetable I wasn't head over heels for. Then I discovered greenhouse-grown eggplants and I was pleasantly surprised! They weren't bitter, so I could eliminate that whole salting process, and they were excellent barbecued. Apparently, tender young eggplants aren't bitter; they only get bitter as they age. Hold the phone, is that a metaphor about life?

2 medium tender young eggplants (about 1½ lb/680 g)

3 cups grape tomatoes, rinsed and drained

2 large cloves garlic, quartered

1 cup chopped fresh cilantro leaves

½ cup (3 oz/85 g) crumbled feta cheese

1 Tbsp extra virgin olive oil

¼ tsp freshly ground black pepper

1 SERVING = 3 ROLL-UPS
PER SERVING: 121 CALORIES, 6.5 G TOTAL FAT, 2.8 G SATURATED FAT, 0 G TRANS FAT, 17 MG CHOLESTEROL, 69 MG SODIUM, 10.6 G CARBOHYDRATE, 3.6 G FIBRE, 4.3 G SUGARS, 0 G ADDED SUGARS, 6.2 G PROTEIN, 336 MG POTASSIUM
CARBOHYDRATE CHOICE = ½ CHOICE

1. Preheat the barbecue to high and make sure your grill is clean. This will prevent the eggplants from sticking, since I don't add any extra oil.

2. While the barbecue is preheating, slice each eggplant lengthwise into nine thin slices. When the barbecue is hot, place the eggplant slices onto the grill, close the lid, and reduce the temperature to medium-high or 400°F.

3. Grill for 3 to 4 minutes on each side, until dark grill marks are visible.

4. Remove the eggplants from the barbecue, place in a bowl, and cover. The steam from the hot eggplants will help soften them so you'll be able to roll them up. Give them a time-out for 15 minutes. Reduce the heat on your barbecue to medium-low or 350°F.

5. While the eggplants are softening, place the tomatoes and garlic into the bowl of a food processor fitted with the steel blade attachment and pulse until roughly chopped. Add the cilantro and gently pulse. Add the crumbled feta and pulse once or twice just to mix it up.

6. Line an 8-inch square metal baking pan with wet parchment paper (see page 15).

7. Lay one piece of eggplant onto a clean counter or cutting board. Place 2 Tbsp tomato filling at the edge closest to you and roll the eggplant up tightly. Place in the prepared pan. Repeat with all the remaining slices.

8. Once the eggplant roll-ups are snug in the pan, drizzle them with the oil and sprinkle with pepper. Place the pan on your barbecue over indirect heat. (If you have a three-burner barbecue, turn off the centre heat source and place the pan there. If you have a two-burner barbecue, turn off one of the heat sources and place the pan there.) Close the lid and cook for 20 to 30 minutes. Check occasionally to make sure the roll-ups aren't burning. When cooked through, remove from the barbecue and let sit for 5 minutes to set before serving. Store any leftovers in the fridge for up to 3 days.

Eggplant Lasagna Stacks VEG GF · *Serves 12*

EGGPLANT IS LOADED WITH SOLUBLE FIBRE. That's the kind that can help regulate blood sugar and reduce cholesterol, which is sadly not so sexy-sounding. I think that's one of the problems with some of the really healthy vegetables—they need pizazz to entice consumers to try them. So, on behalf of eggplants everywhere, I've appointed myself as their PR rep. Here's my spin: "Change up your lasagna. Give pasta the day off and use gorgeous white and aubergine strips instead. Your guests will be begging you for the recipe!"

2 medium tender young eggplants (about 1½ lb/680 g)

2 large red, yellow, or orange peppers, seeds removed and cut in quarters

1 cup low-fat ricotta

1 cup (3 oz/85 g) grated Parmigiano-Reggiano

12 large fresh basil leaves

1 (19 fl oz/540 mL) can diced tomatoes, petite cut, flavoured or plain

2 large cloves garlic, crushed

1 SERVING = 1 STACK
PER SERVING: 63 CALORIES, 2 G TOTAL FAT,
1.1 G SATURATED FAT, 0 G TRANS FAT,
8 MG CHOLESTEROL, 76 MG SODIUM,
8.5 G CARBOHYDRATE, 2.5 G FIBRE,
4.3 G SUGARS, 0 G ADDED SUGARS,
3.7 G PROTEIN, 314 MG POTASSIUM
CARBOHYDRATE CHOICE = < 1 CHOICE

1. Preheat the barbecue to high. Rinse and pat dry the eggplants. Cut each eggplant lengthwise into 12 thin slices. Place the eggplants on the barbecue, close the lid, and reduce the temperature to medium-high (400°F).

2. Grill the eggplants for 3 to 5 minutes and then flip over. Close the lid. Grill another 3 to 5 minutes, until softer but not dried out. Transfer the slices to a plate.

3. Grill the peppers for 5 to 8 minutes per side with the barbecue lid closed.

4. Line a 9 × 13-inch metal baking dish with wet parchment paper (see page 15), making sure all the edges are folded in.

5. Place 12 slices of the roasted eggplant in the bottom of the dish.

6. Mix the ricotta and Parmigiano-Reggiano together in a medium bowl. Top each of the eggplant slices with equal amounts of the cheese mixture.

7. Coarsely chop the grilled peppers and sprinkle over top of the cheese. Top each eggplant slice with one basil leaf, then top with the remaining 12 slices of eggplant.

8. Mix together the canned tomatoes and crushed garlic. Evenly pour over top.

9. Place the baking dish in your barbecue over indirect heat. (If you have a three-burner barbecue, turn off the centre burner; if you have a two-burner barbecue, turn off one side. Place the pan over the area that is turned off.) Close the lid and cook for 25 to 30 minutes until warmed throughout. If you don't have a barbecue, bake in the oven at 350°F for 25 to 30 minutes.

10. Remove from the barbecue and let sit for 10 minutes, then serve.

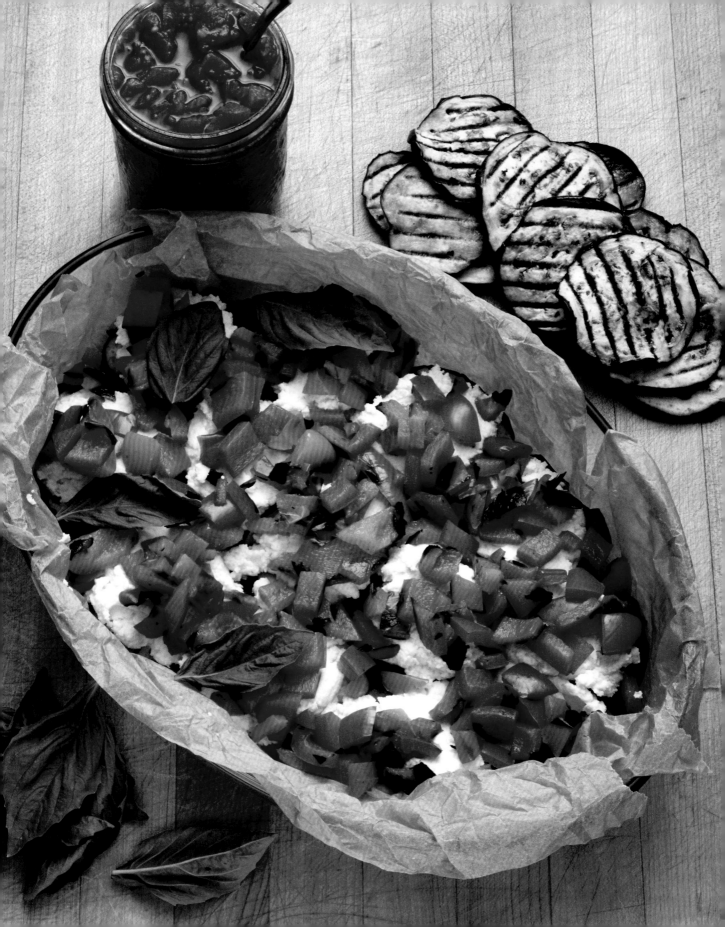

Stir-Fried Brussels Sprouts with Bacon & Cranberries LF · *Serves 6*

BRUSSELS SPROUTS ARE ONE OF THE MOST MALIGNED VEGETABLES to take up residence in the produce department from mid-September through December. I believe if you have just one grey-blob Brussels sprout experience, it scars your taste buds for life. My husband, Scott, had such an experience, but this recipe turned him from an abstainer into a believer. All it took was bacon and maple syrup.

2 oz (56 g) diced low-sodium bacon (see note)

3 shallots, finely chopped

1 lb (450 g) Brussels sprouts, trimmed and thinly sliced

½ cup fresh or frozen cranberries

2 Tbsp apple cider vinegar

1 Tbsp pure amber maple syrup

¼ tsp table salt

NOTE: Low-sodium bacon? Yes, there is such a product; you can find it with the other bacon.

1. Heat a large 12- or 14-inch skillet over medium-high heat. Add the bacon and sauté until golden brown and slightly crispy, 3 to 5 minutes.

2. Add the shallots, reduce heat to medium, and sauté until golden brown, 4 to 6 minutes.

3. Add the Brussels sprouts, cranberries, and vinegar; sauté until well combined, then cover and reduce heat to medium-low. Cook for 2 to 4 minutes, until the sprouts are a fabulous dark green. Please don't overcook them; we are trying to avoid grey blobs of overcooked Brussels sprouts!

4. Remove the lid, drizzle with the maple syrup, and sauté for 30 seconds. Sprinkle with the salt and serve.

1 SERVING = ½ CUP
PER SERVING: 99 CALORIES, 4 G TOTAL FAT, 1.3 G SATURATED FAT, 0 G TRANS FAT, 9 MG CHOLESTEROL, 192 MG SODIUM, 13.6 G CARBOHYDRATE, 4.2 G FIBRE, 4.2 G SUGARS, 2 G ADDED SUGARS, 4.2 G PROTEIN, 428 MG POTASSIUM
CARBOHYDRATE CHOICE = 1 CHOICE

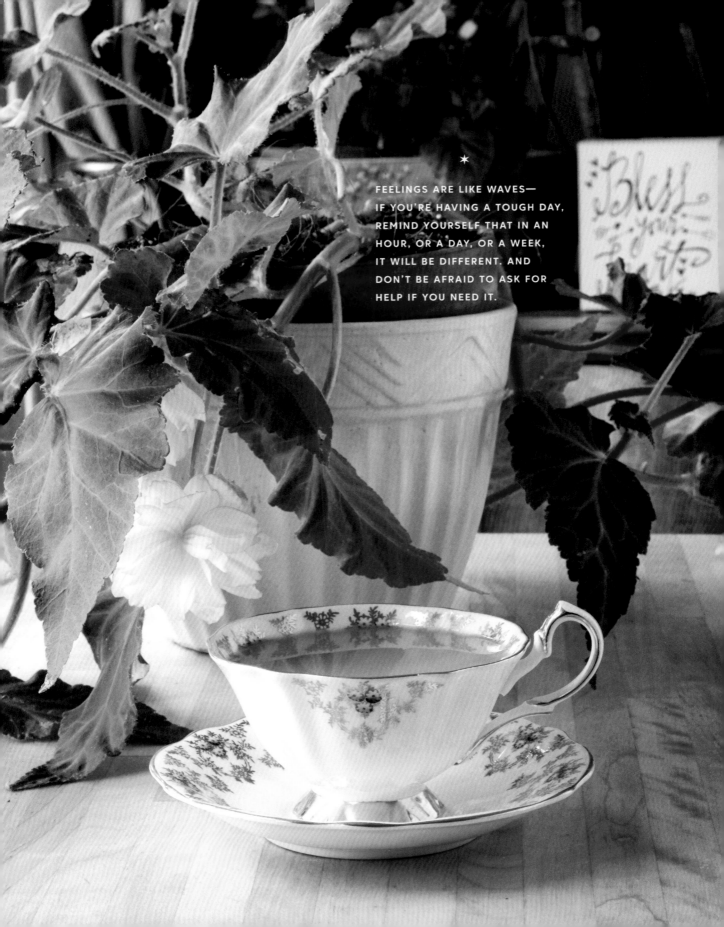

FEELINGS ARE LIKE WAVES—
IF YOU'RE HAVING A TOUGH DAY,
REMIND YOURSELF THAT IN AN
HOUR, OR A DAY, OR A WEEK,
IT WILL BE DIFFERENT. AND
DON'T BE AFRAID TO ASK FOR
HELP IF YOU NEED IT.

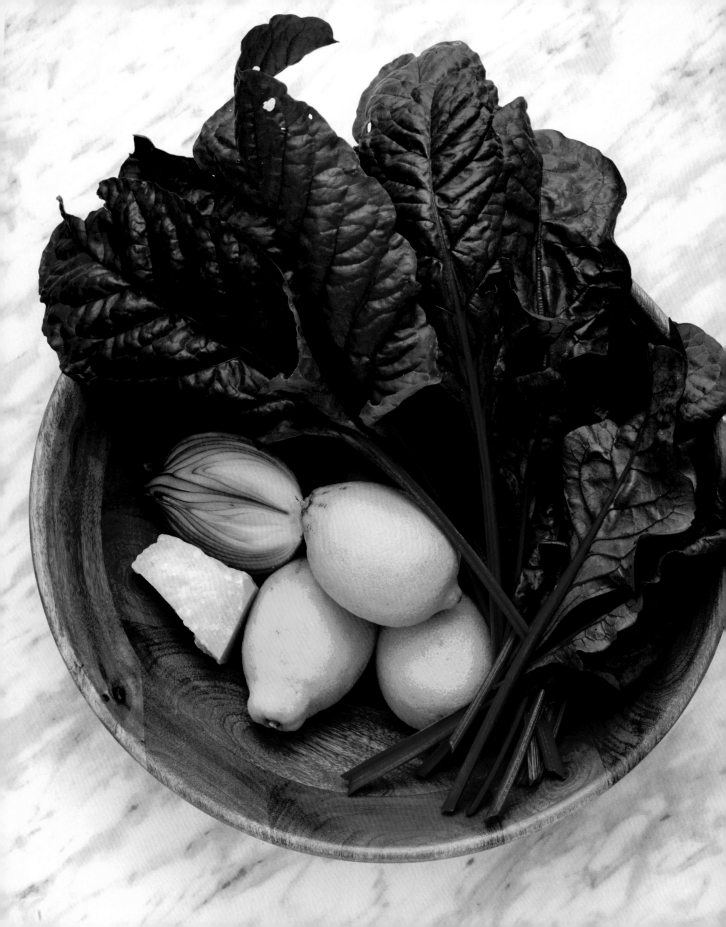

Swiss Chard with Lemon & Pecorino VEG GF · *Serves 4*

MOST YEARS I GROW SWISS CHARD IN MY KITCHEN GARDEN IN A LARGE WHISKY BARREL. Whenever I want a quick and easy summer side dish, I just walk out my back door and pick some. I know that most people don't have Swiss chard growing in their backyards in whisky barrels, so this recipe calls for one bunch, the way it is sold in grocery stores.

1 Tbsp canola oil

¾ cup thinly sliced red onion

1 large clove garlic, minced

1 bunch Swiss chard, stems removed, sliced into 1-inch ribbons (see note)

1 Tbsp fresh lemon juice

2 Tbsp grated Pecorino Romano

1. Heat a 12- or 14-inch non-stick skillet over medium heat. Add the oil and red onion and sauté for 1 to 2 minutes, until the onion starts to soften. Add the garlic and Swiss chard and sauté until the chard wilts, 1 to 3 minutes.

2. Add the lemon juice, sprinkle with Pecorino Romano, and quickly combine. Serve right away.

NOTE: Swiss chard is very much like spinach in the shrinkage category—a whole lot of raw shrinks down to a small amount when cooked. Feel free to double the recipe, but remember that you'll need a bigger skillet.

1 SERVING = ¼ CUP
PER SERVING: 87 CALORIES, 4.7 G TOTAL FAT, 0.9 G SATURATED FAT, 0 G TRANS FAT, 4 MG CHOLESTEROL, 234 MG SODIUM, 9.8 G CARBOHYDRATE, 2.5 G FIBRE, 3.8 G SUGARS, 0 G ADDED SUGARS, 3.3 G PROTEIN, 433 MG POTASSIUM
CARBOHYDRATE CHOICE = ½ CHOICE

Lemon Barley Pilaf LF · *Serves 6 to 8*

TO BE ABLE TO WRITE A HEALTH CLAIM ON A LABEL takes years of research and scientific documentation. When you see this on a label—"barley fibre helps reduce/lower cholesterol"—bear in mind that it probably is easier to complete an Ironman than to get permission from Health Canada or the U.S. Food and Drug Administration to include that claim on your label. Science and research aside, one bite of this pilaf and you won't even be thinking about health claims. You'll just be wondering if there is any more.

1 Tbsp canola oil

1 onion, diced

4 cloves garlic, diced

1 cup pot barley, rinsed and well drained

2 cups no-salt-added chicken broth

⅓ cup minced fresh parsley leaves

Zest of 2 lemons (2 to 3 Tbsp) (see note)

3 Tbsp capers, rinsed, drained, and coarsely chopped

⅛ tsp table salt

NOTE: I love the taste of lemon, but a couple of my taste testers felt it was too lemony. I'm letting you be the Keeper of the Lemoniness. Love lemons? Go with the full 3 Tbsp. Like lemons? Go with 2 Tbsp.

1. Place a 3½-quart or large saucepan over medium heat. Add the oil and sauté the onion until it starts to turn golden, 3 to 5 minutes. Add the garlic and sauté for about 1 minute. Add the barley and sauté for another minute to lightly toast it.

2. Pour in the broth. Bring to a boil, then stir, cover, reduce heat to a simmer, and cook for 25 to 30 minutes. Check the pot at 15 minutes; if the pot is almost dry, then reduce the heat. If it's still a big soupy mess, raise the heat slightly. The barley is cooked when 99% of the liquid is absorbed. It shouldn't be mushy or dry and burnt. Perfectly cooked barley should be slightly chewy.

3. When the barley is cooked, remove the pot from the heat and fluff it with a fork. Let sit, covered, for 5 minutes to help redistribute all of the liquid and produce a fluffier barley dish.

4. Add the parsley, zest, capers, and salt, lightly mix in, and serve. You can make this the day before and serve it as a cold salad.

1 SERVING = ½ CUP
PER SERVING: 118 CALORIES, 2.4 G TOTAL FAT, 0.3 G SATURATED FAT, 0 G TRANS FAT, 0 MG CHOLESTEROL, 267 MG SODIUM, 21.1 G CARBOHYDRATE, 4.9 G FIBRE, 1 G SUGARS, 0 G ADDED SUGARS, 4.3 G PROTEIN, 172 MG POTASSIUM
CARBOHYDRATE CHOICE = 1 CHOICE

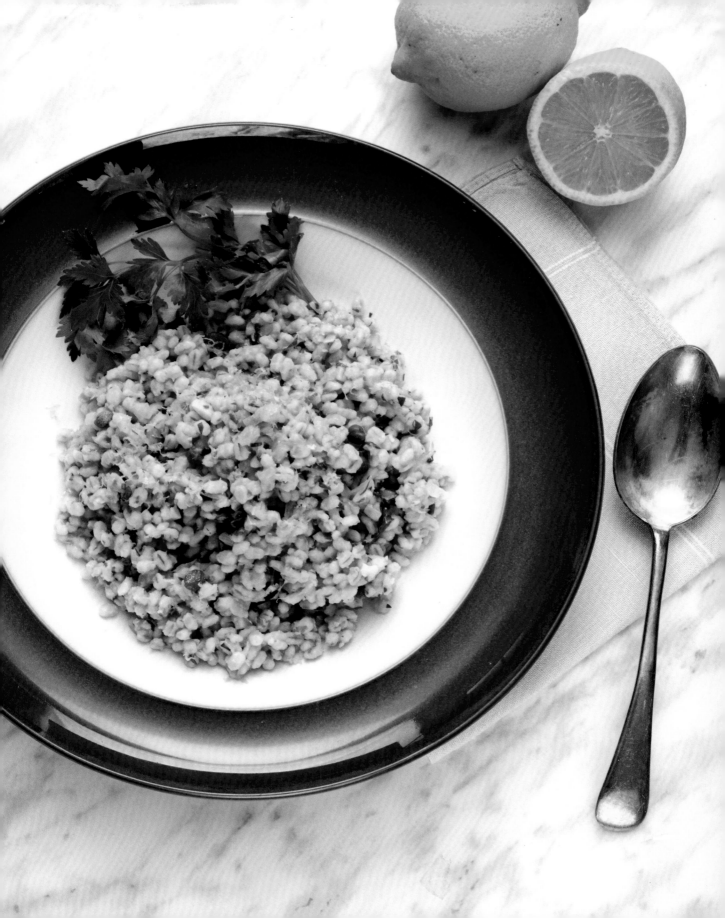

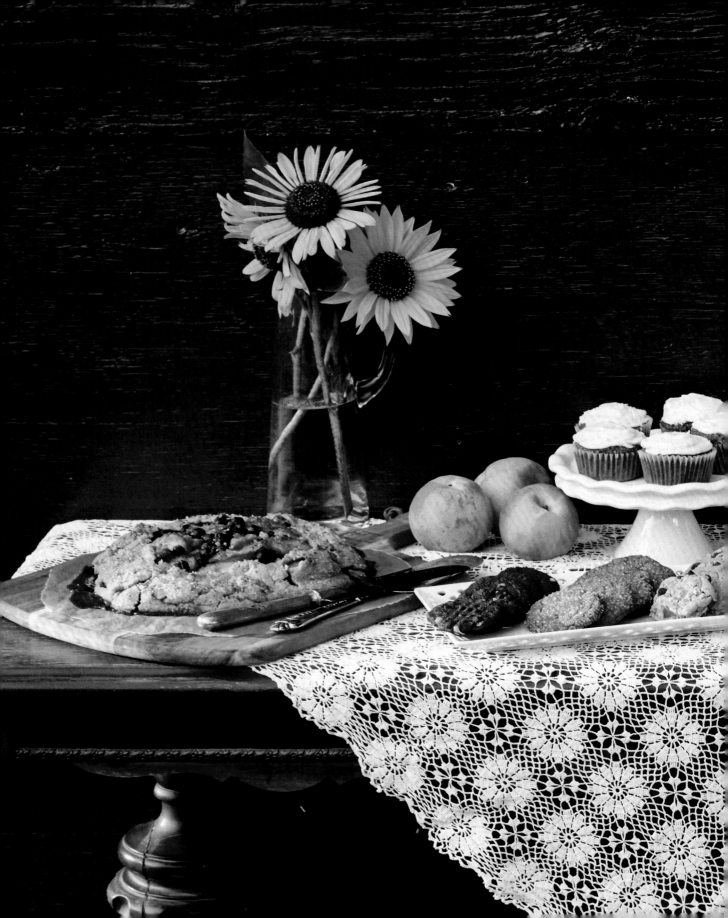

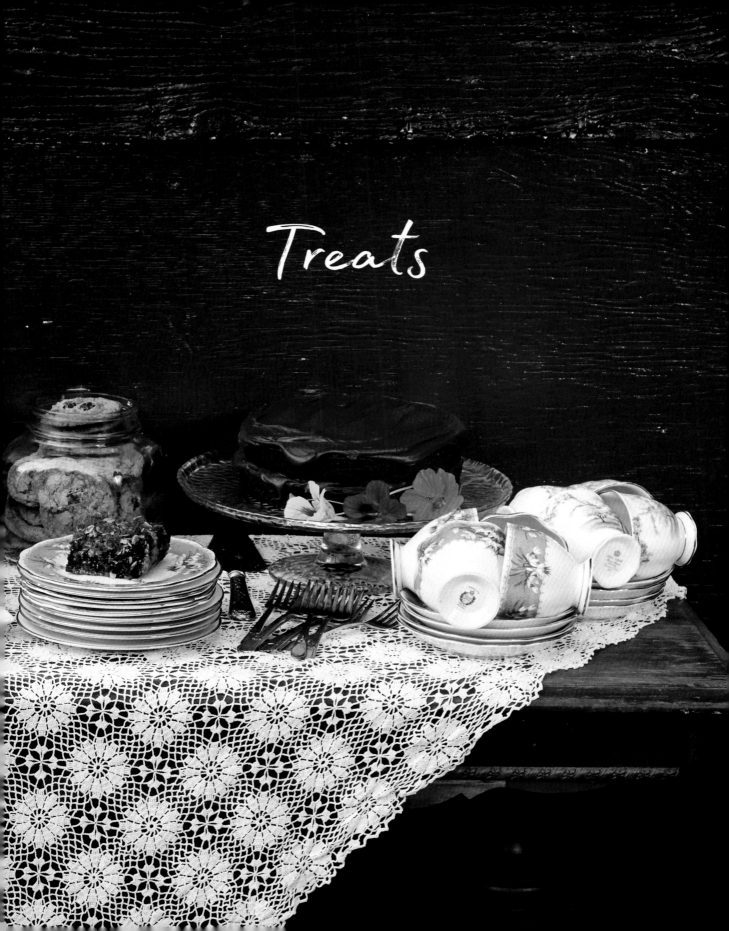

Treats

You say "dessert,"
I say "treat."

Do you remember the
word *treat*?

As in, "If you've been
really, really good, you can
have a *treat*."

As in, "Wow, that's extraordinary!
Congratulations! Let's celebrate!
Let's have a *treat*."

As in, "It's your birthday,
here's a huge piece of cake—it's a *treat*."

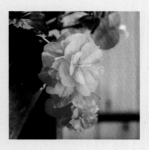

Some people call treats "dessert." Say "dessert" at my house and you're probably getting sliced peaches, chunks of watermelon, frozen grapes, or a citrus fruit salad. Say "treat" at my house and you'll be getting a slice of my Chocolate Fudge Cake (page 219), or a wedge of Peach & Blueberry Galette (page 211), or one of the other fabulous treats in this chapter.

Treats are part of our lives, and I'm all for them—I don't look at them as a forbidden food. However, in recent years, people have begun to eat treats all day in lieu of healthy, delicious foods. And therein lies the problem. Treats are not evil. But the frequency of those treats can lead to some health issues. So, say yes to treats, but remember to keep them for special occasions and enjoy every single bite with abandon.

Baking & Cookie Rules

BAKING IS A SCIENCE. Without the right ingredients and the proper techniques, your baked goods can be a complete disaster. Here's my list of rules (based on the fan emails that I've received) that will help you bake a perfect muffin or biscuit, cake, square, or cookie every time.

1. Make sure your oven is calibrated. Just because your oven dial says the temperature is 325°F doesn't mean that's the temperature in the oven. Buy a thermometer that you hang on the rack and check to see if your oven is registering the correct temperature. If the recipe says 325°F and your new thermometer says 300°F, then you need to adjust.

2. Most baked goods bake better when the rack is in the middle of the oven. If the rack is too high, the tops of your treats will bake faster than the bottoms. If the rack is too low, the bottoms will cook faster than the tops.

3. When it comes to cookies, don't use a thermal baking sheet or a rimmed baking sheet. Cookies love being baked on a rimless baking sheet, preferably a light, shiny one. Rimmed baking sheets keep the air from circulating evenly around the cookies as they bake. Rimless baking sheets allow the air to flow around perfectly.

4. Line pans with parchment paper if you hate washing dishes as much as I do, or if you don't want to add any extra fat to the recipe by greasing the pan. I use wet parchment in some recipes and dry in others. Check the instructions.

5. There are two types of measuring cups: the type for dry ingredients like flour, sugar, and wheat germ, and the type for liquids like water, oil, and milk. See the picture on page 188 to learn the difference.

6. I use canola oil in most of my heart-healthy baking. You need to measure oil for baking in a glass or see-through measuring cup. Pour in the oil at eye level so the bottom of the meniscus is at the correct measurement. Using the wrong type of measuring cup will totally wreck the recipes. See page 188.

7. When you are packing brown sugar, you must go back to your childhood and channel your sandcastle-making skills. Remember that if you didn't pack the sand in tight enough, the castle would crumble, there'd be tears, and the day was ruined. You don't have to go all Herculean on me, but pack the brown sugar in.

8. Too much or too little flour can spell disaster for any baked goods, but especially for my recipes, because they use whole grain flours. Make sure to measure all whole grain flours correctly using this method: spoon flour into a dry measuring cup so it's heaping, then use a straight-edged spatula to level it off. I did the science experiments, and improper measuring can result in as much as a ¼-cup difference. In the baking world, that's huge. See the picture on page 188.

9. Ground flaxseed and flaxseed meal are different. Most of my baking recipes call for flaxseed meal; it's finer and blends better in the batter (oh, how I love alliteration). See page 184 for my Flaxseed Tutorial.

10. Use ice-cream scoops with a release button to make sure all the cookies and muffins are the same size. They come in a range of sizes. Check to make sure you are using the correct size. See a picture of all my scoops on page 189.

High-Fibre Baking Pantry

Measuring Cups, Both Dry and Wet

Glass or transparent measuring cups are for liquids. The plastic or metal non-transparent ones are for dry ingredients or ingredients that are extremely thick, like peanut butter. See a picture on the facing page.

Using the correct measuring tool is important. A carpenter doesn't measure a large piece of drywall board with a small wooden ruler, so don't measure a cup of milk in a dry measuring cup designed for flour.

1% Buttermilk

In Canada, buttermilk is made using 1% milk, though occasionally you can find it with 2% to 3% fat. If you don't have any buttermilk kicking around your fridge, do not fear, I've got the solution. If the recipe calls for 1 cup 1% buttermilk, pour 1 Tbsp apple cider vinegar, white vinegar, or fresh lemon juice into a 1-cup glass measuring cup. Add 1% milk until you reach the 1-cup mark on the measuring cup. Make sure you are reading the cup at eye level. The milk will start to curdle, but don't worry—it's supposed to. Stir and use in your recipe.

Dark Brown Sugar

Dark brown sugar, sometimes called old-fashioned sugar, adds a great flavour and colour to baked goods. Demerara sugar is not the same as dark brown sugar. Demerara is very coarse and has a stronger flavour, and it doesn't bake up the same way.

Coarse or Sanding Sugar

This is larger than your regular granulated sugar. When sprinkled on baked goods before they head into the oven, it adds sparkle, sweetness, and a crunch to the finished product.

Flaxseed Tutorial

If I created a Kingdom of Fibre, I would appoint flaxseed to be the King. This tiny little seed has a five-pointed crown because it contains:

- heart-healthy omega-3 fatty acids
- both types of fibre: soluble and insoluble
- plant lignans that have two outstanding properties: they act as a phytoestrogen that appears to lower your chances of breast and prostate cancer, and they have antioxidant properties that help protect your cells against heart disease

Flaxseed, both brown and golden, is widely available in larger grocery stores, with many choices:

- Whole flaxseed. You'll need to grind this up in a coffee grinder. Whole seeds can be stored in a cool, dark place for up to one year.
- Ground flaxseed. This is already ground for you. Store it in your fridge for up to three months or freeze it for a longer shelf life.
- Flaxseed meal or milled flaxseed. Although there isn't a regulation for how fine flaxseed meal is compared to ground flaxseed, I have found that, depending on the brand, flaxseed meal (or milled flaxseed) is very finely ground and is perfect for some of the baking recipes in this cookbook. If you don't want to buy this kind of flaxseed, grind up whole seeds yourself until they are very finely ground.

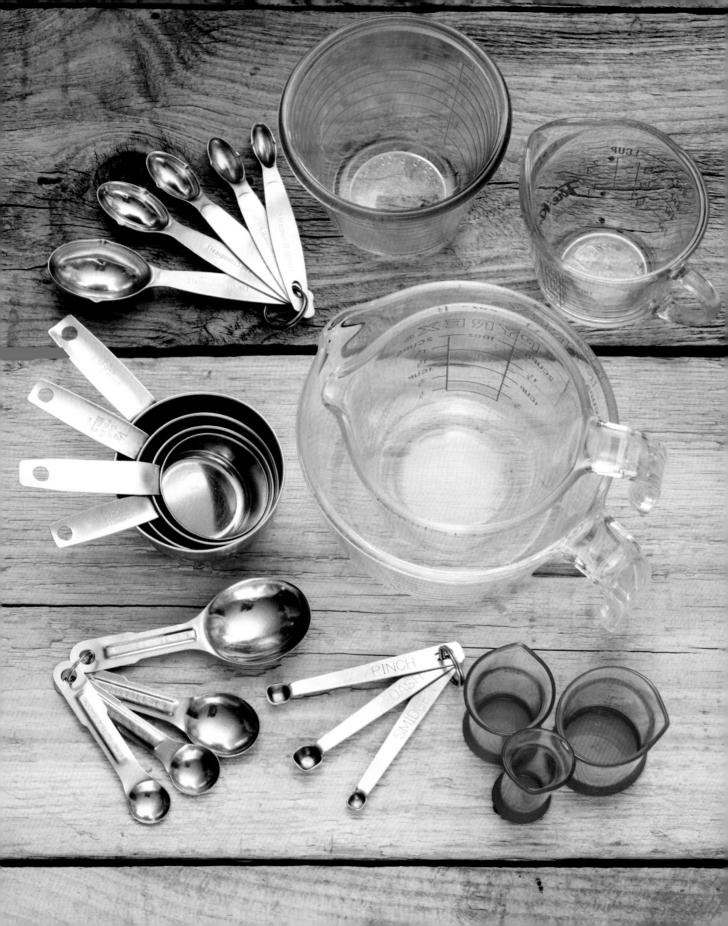

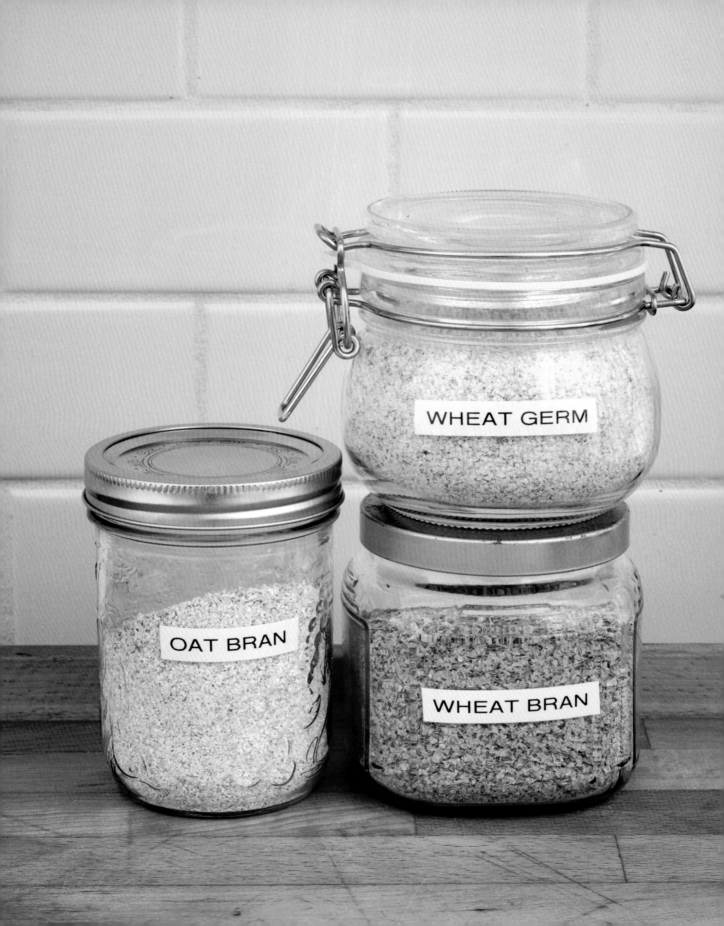

- Roasted whole flaxseed. Fee Fi Fo Flax, a company out of Saskatchewan, roasts their golden flaxseed, which gives it a nutty flavour and eliminates the need for grinding. The hard outer layer is slightly broken down, making the nutrients in the flaxseed available without grinding.

Natural Cocoa Powder

Natural cocoa powder is higher in flavanols (those powerful antioxidants that can help reduce your blood pressure) than regular cocoa powder. Regular cocoa powder may be labelled as "Dutch process." Dutching destroys nearly two-thirds of those powerful antioxidants. I use only natural or raw cocoa powder in all my recipes, and I'll ask you to do the same. When shopping, read the front of the package or container. Look for "natural," "natural unsweetened," or "raw cacao."

Flours

WHOLE WHEAT FLOUR

Don't let the "whole" part fool you. Whole wheat flour is not the whole wheat kernel. When a whole grain wheat kernel is milled, the outer bran as well as the fatty germ are removed, leaving you with all-purpose flour. Add the bran back and you have whole wheat. The problem is, the germ has not been added back. To make whole wheat flour whole grain whole wheat, I add wheat germ to recipes. If you can find stone-milled whole wheat flour, that's the real deal.

BARLEY FLOUR

Barley flour is made from whole grain barley and contains both cholesterol-lowering soluble fibre and GI tract–moving insoluble fibre. I use barley flour in most of the baking in this cookbook because it adds so much extra fibre. It contains gluten, so it works well in my baking. The milling process doesn't change the quality of the soluble flour, which means it's still a great source of those powerful beta-glucans that aid in lowering cholesterol. I buy my barley flour at a bulk food store.

OAT FLOUR

Oat flour is also high in fibre, but it does not contain gluten. However, depending on where it was grown or processed, the oat flour may have traces of gluten. If you are living with celiac disease, look for certified gluten-free oats, oat flour, and oat bran. You can make your own whole grain oat flour by grinding large oat flakes in a food processor.

Natural Wheat Germ

The germ of any whole grain is where germination starts. It contains most of the good-for-you nutrients, including B vitamins, heart-healthy fat, trace minerals, and vitamin E. Natural wheat germ is not toasted and can be found in bags near the hot cereal section of a grocery store. Because it contains fat, wheat germ should be stored in the fridge for up to three months or in the freezer for up to six months.

Oat & Wheat Bran

Both are the outer portion of a whole grain and contain fibre. Oat bran is often sold as "oat bran creamy hot cereal."

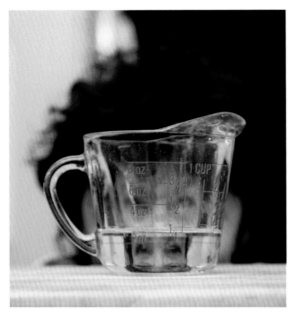

MEASURING LIQUIDS: Lower yourself down to eye level and look for the meniscus.

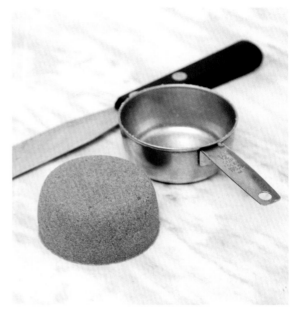

MEASURING BROWN SUGAR: Pat it down firmly in cup, and level off using a spatula.

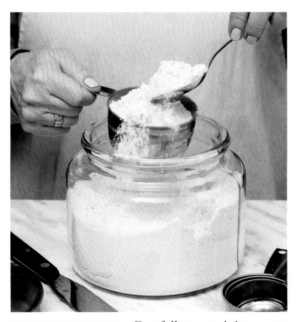

MEASURING FLOUR: Carefully spoon it into a cup.

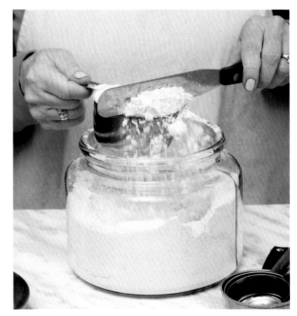

Level off using a spatula.

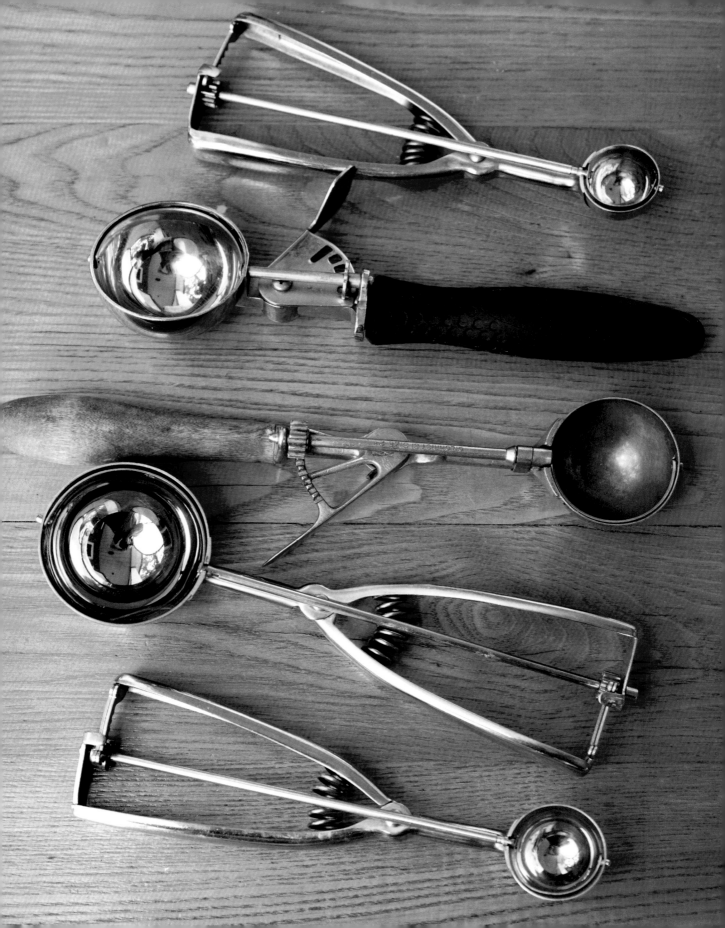

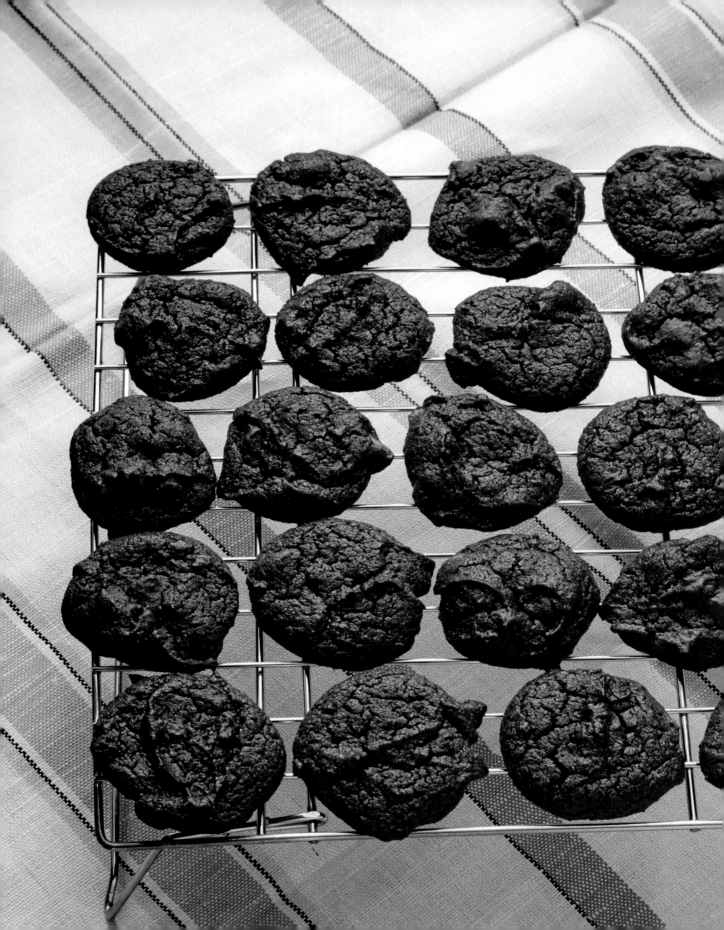

Chocolate Fudgy Brownie Bites VEG GF · *Makes 40 (2-inch) cookies*

OH, THE PERILS OF RECIPE DEVELOPING. The warm spring day when I was developing these chocolate morsels, a squirrel, who I expect was tempted by the heavenly chocolate wafting through my screen door, somehow pried his way into my kitchen while I was upstairs in my office. I was busy writing up the recipe when I heard some odd noises coming from downstairs. I walked in to find the culprit on a chocolate high and having a heyday with an entire cookie in his mouth. The place was a wreck of chocolate crumbs and half-eaten cookies. On a positive note, these cookies are gluten-free and apparently squirrel-approved.

¼ cup + 2 Tbsp canola oil
(see page 183)

2 Tbsp liquid honey

¾ cup packed dark brown sugar

¼ cup flaxseed meal
(see page 184)

1 omega-3 egg

1 Tbsp pure vanilla extract

½ cup natural cocoa powder

¾ cup + 1 Tbsp whole grain oat
flour (see page 187)

¼ tsp baking soda

¼ cup dark or bittersweet
chocolate chips

1. Place a rack in the middle of your oven and preheat the oven to 375°F. Line two rimless baking sheets with parchment paper.

2. In a medium bowl, using a hand-held electric mixer or a wooden spoon, beat together the oil, honey, and brown sugar until it looks like wet sand, 2 to 4 minutes.

3. Add the flaxseed meal, egg, and vanilla and beat until thick and creamy and a lighter shade of brown, 1 to 3 minutes.

4. Add the cocoa powder and gently beat in on low speed (if using a mixer). Don't beat on high, or you'll be wearing cocoa powder when it flies out of the bowl and lands on your clothes (I know from experience). When the cocoa powder is totally incorporated, beat for an additional minute. Add the flour and baking soda and gently beat to combine. Add the chocolate chips and stir in well.

5. Using a 2-teaspoon ice-cream scoop with a release button, measure out and drop the dough onto one of the prepared pans. You should get 20 scoops onto one sheet.

6. Bake the cookies for 8 to 9 minutes until the tops crack, then remove from the oven and let rest on the baking sheet for 3 minutes. Remove and let cool completely on a wire cooling rack. Finish baking the rest of the dough.

7. Store cooled cookies in a covered container for up to 1 week or freeze for up to 3 months.

1 SERVING = 2 COOKIES
PER SERVING: 128 CALORIES, 6.7 G TOTAL FAT, 1.2 G SATURATED FAT, 0 G TRANS FAT,
10 MG CHOLESTEROL, 11 MG SODIUM, 17 G CARBOHYDRATE, 2 G FIBRE, 12.4 G SUGARS,
11.7 G ADDED SUGARS, 1.4 G PROTEIN, 85 G POTASSIUM
CARBOHYDRATE CHOICE = 1 CHOICE

Decadent Chocolate Chunk Cookies VEG · *Makes 34 (3-inch) cookies*

THESE RICH, BUTTERY, DECADENT COOKIES are loaded with chocolate and are perfect for a special occasion. Say you win the Nobel Peace Prize, your adult child gets a job in their chosen profession, or you win a lottery—you get the drift. These cookies are a treat, my friend. I repeat, a treat.

6 oz (170 g) dark or bittersweet chocolate (see note)

1½ cups whole grain barley flour

¼ cup flaxseed meal (see page 184)

1 tsp baking soda

½ cup unsalted butter, room temperature

¾ cup packed dark brown sugar

¼ cup granulated sugar

1 omega-3 egg

2 tsp pure vanilla extract

NOTE: What does 6 oz (170 g) of chopped dark or bittersweet chocolate look like if you don't have a scale? That would be 1¼ cups.

1. Place a rack in the middle of your oven and preheat the oven to 350°F. Line a rimless baking sheet with parchment paper.

2. Using a butcher's knife or a paring knife, pierce the chocolate to make chunks. I prefer a mixture of both large (as in a blueberry) and small (as in a pea) pieces, but it's your call. Set aside.

3. In a medium bowl, whisk together the flour, flaxseed meal, and baking soda.

4. In a large bowl, using a hand-held electric mixer, cream the butter until wispy little horns appear on the edge of the beaters and the butter is a paler shade of yellow. Add the brown sugar and beat until well incorporated, 2 to 3 minutes. Add the granulated sugar and beat to combine, 2 to 3 minutes. Add the egg and vanilla and beat until the mixture turns a lighter beige. Add the flour mixture and gently stir in. Fold in the chocolate chunks.

5. Using a 1-tablespoon ice-cream scoop with a release button, measure out and drop the dough onto the baking sheet, making sure that the cookies are at least 1 inch apart. I put 12 cookies per baking sheet, because these cookies really spread out. You'll need to bake these in batches.

6. Bake for 10 to 11 minutes until crispy-looking. They will be very flat. Remove the cookies from the oven and let them sit on the baking sheet for about 4 minutes, until they have set. Transfer to a wire rack to finish cooling. Bake the rest of the dough. They taste better cooled, so practise the art of delayed gratification and wait at least 30 minutes. Store in an airtight container for up to 2 days or freeze them for up to 2 months.

1 SERVING = 2 COOKIES
PER SERVING: 212 CALORIES, 10.7 G TOTAL FAT, 6.1 G SATURATED FAT, 0 G TRANS FAT, 26 MG CHOLESTEROL, 87 MG SODIUM, 26.3 G CARBOHYDRATE, 3.5 G FIBRE, 17.1 G SUGARS, 15.4 G ADDED SUGARS, 1.2 G PROTEIN, 147 MG POTASSIUM
CARBOHYDRATE CHOICE = 1½ CHOICES

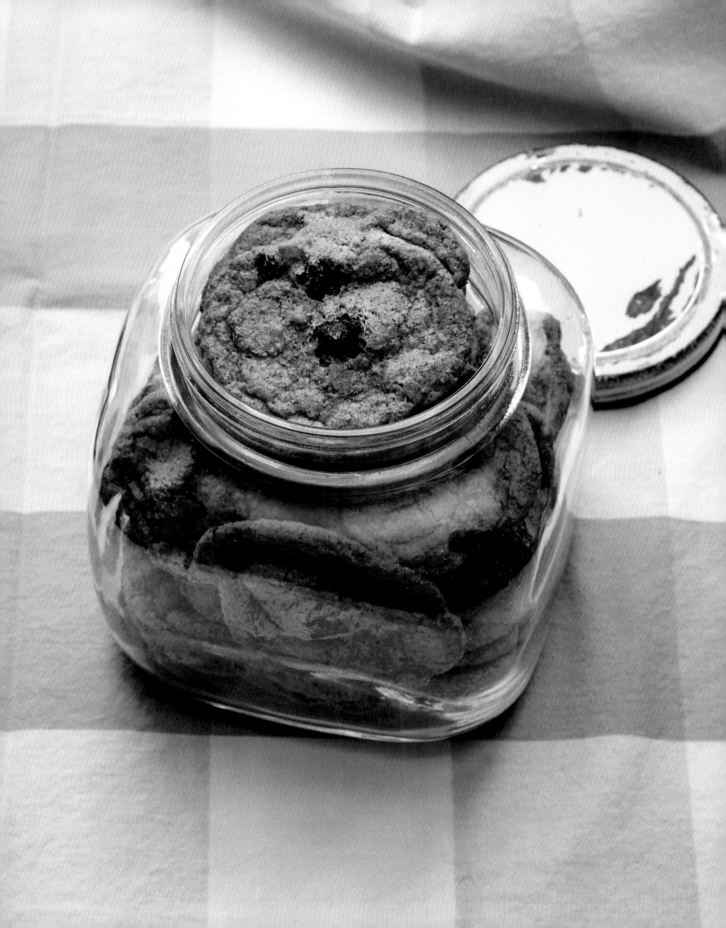

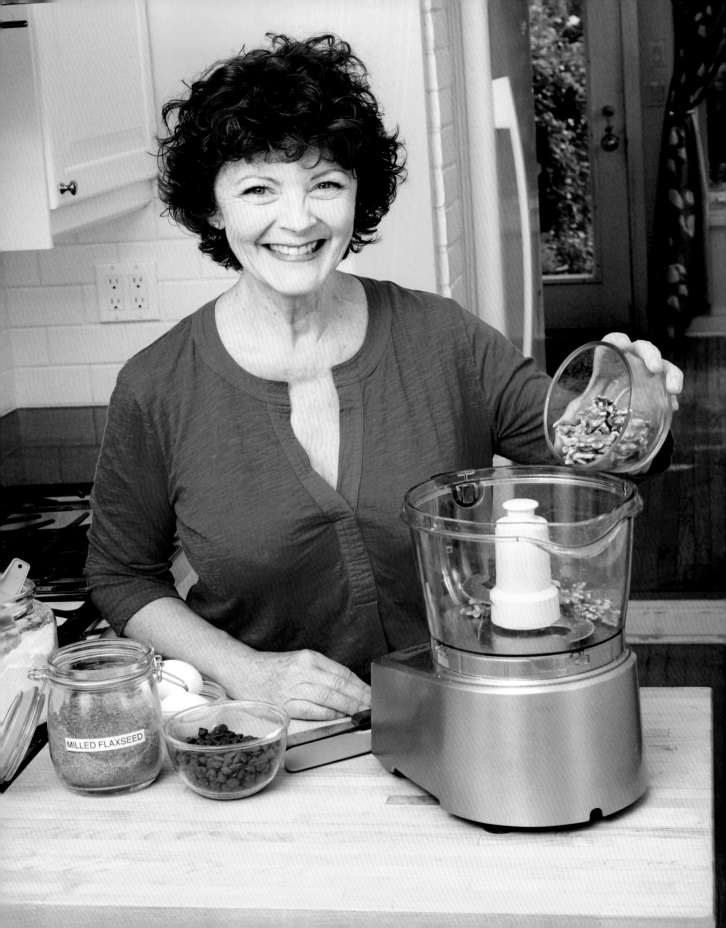

Walnut Flaxseed Transformer Cookies   VEG · *Makes 44 (1½-inch) cookies*

HAVE YOU EVER BEEN SITTING ON YOUR COUCH, channel surfing, when suddenly you get an overwhelming desire for chocolate? It was 8 p.m., there was nothing on TV, and out of the blue my inner chocoholic whispered, "You MUST bake with chocolate." I did a mental scan of my pantry (no sense hauling my sorry butt off the couch for nothing), and 30 minutes later I had a cookie that was a cross between an Italian amaretti (minus the almonds) and a regular cookie with hints of chocolate and nuts in every bite. The first day you make these, they are slightly crunchy, and by day three, they miraculously transform themselves into something like biscotti. Hence the name: Transformer Cookies.

1 cup whole walnuts

1 cup dark or bittersweet chocolate chips

1 cup whole grain barley flour

1 cup flaxseed meal (see page 184)

2 omega-3 eggs

1 cup granulated sugar

1 tsp pure vanilla extract

1. Place an oven rack in the middle of the oven and preheat the oven to 350°F. Line a rimless baking sheet with parchment paper. Set aside.

2. Place the walnuts and chocolate chips into the bowl of a food processor fitted with the steel blade attachment, and pulse until they are finely ground, but not a paste. Add the flour and pulse just until the flour has been well distributed. Add the flaxseed meal and pulse gently. Set aside.

3. In a large bowl, using a hand-held electric mixer, beat the eggs until frothy, about 45 seconds. Add the sugar ¼ cup at a time, beating well between additions. You are pumping in air as you beat, and this helps make the cookies fabulous. This should take 4 to 6 minutes total. Patience, my friend, it's worth it. The cookies are counting on you.

4. Once all the sugar has been added, beat in the vanilla. Then, using a rubber spatula, gently fold in the walnut-chocolate mixture until well combined. Make sure not to overmix.

5. Using a 2-teaspoon ice-cream scoop with a release button, measure out and drop the dough onto the prepared pan. You should get 22 teaspoonfuls. Dampen your finger and slightly press down on the tops of the cookies. Bake for 13 to 15 minutes, until they are crispy looking. Let cool on the baking sheet for 2 minutes, then transfer to a wire rack to finish cooling. Repeat with the remaining dough. Once cooled, store the cookies in an airtight container for up to 2 weeks or freeze for up to 3 months.

1 SERVING = 2 COOKIES
PER SERVING: 177 CALORIES, 9.2 G TOTAL FAT, 2.5 G SATURATED FAT, 0 G TRANS FAT, 18 MG CHOLESTEROL, 8 MG SODIUM, 22.8 G CARBOHYDRATE, 3.4 G FIBRE, 15.9 G SUGARS, 15.6 G ADDED SUGARS, 3.5 G PROTEIN, 120 MG POTASSIUM
CARBOHYDRATE CHOICE = 1 CHOICE

Oatmeal Chocolate Chip Cookies VEG GF · *Makes 20 (4-inch) cookies*

I LOVE HOW A CERTAIN FOOD OR COOKING AROMA can transport you back in time to a specific place. These cookies take me back to my gran's kitchen. Granny made a fabulous oatmeal cookie, and I added the chocolate, because, well hello, I'm a card-carrying chocoholic.

½ cup canola oil (see page 183)

¾ cup packed dark brown sugar

1 omega-3 egg

1 Tbsp pure vanilla extract

1¼ cups whole grain oat flour (see page 187)

1 cup large oat flakes (see note)

¼ cup oat bran

½ tsp baking soda

¼ cup gluten-free dark or bittersweet chocolate chips

NOTE: To make these gluten-free, use oat flour and large oat flakes that are labelled "gluten-free."

1. Place a rack in the middle of your oven and preheat the oven to 375°F. Line a rimless baking sheet with parchment paper.

2. In a medium bowl, using a hand-held electric mixer, beat the oil and brown sugar until it looks like wet sand, 2 to 3 minutes.

3. Add the egg and vanilla and beat until thick and creamy, 1 to 2 minutes.

4. Add the flour, oat flakes, oat bran, and baking soda and gently beat until combined. Add the chocolate chips and stir in well.

5. Using a 2-tablespoon ice-cream scoop with a release button, measure out and drop the dough onto the prepared baking sheet. You should get about 10 on one baking sheet.

6. Bake for 11 to 12 minutes, until golden brown. Remove the cookies from the oven and let sit on the baking sheet for 4 minutes to set. Transfer the cookies to a wire rack to finish cooling. Finish baking the rest of the dough.

7. Store the cooled cookies in a covered container for up to 1 week or freeze for up to 3 months.

1 SERVING = 1 COOKIE
PER SERVING: 165 CALORIES, 7.7 G TOTAL FAT, 1.1 G SATURATED FAT, 0 G TRANS FAT, 10 MG CHOLESTEROL, 38 MG SODIUM, 21.3 G CARBOHYDRATE, 2 G FIBRE, 9.4 G SUGARS, 9.4 G ADDED SUGARS, 3.5 G PROTEIN, 88 MG POTASSIUM
CARBOHYDRATE CHOICE = 1 CHOICE

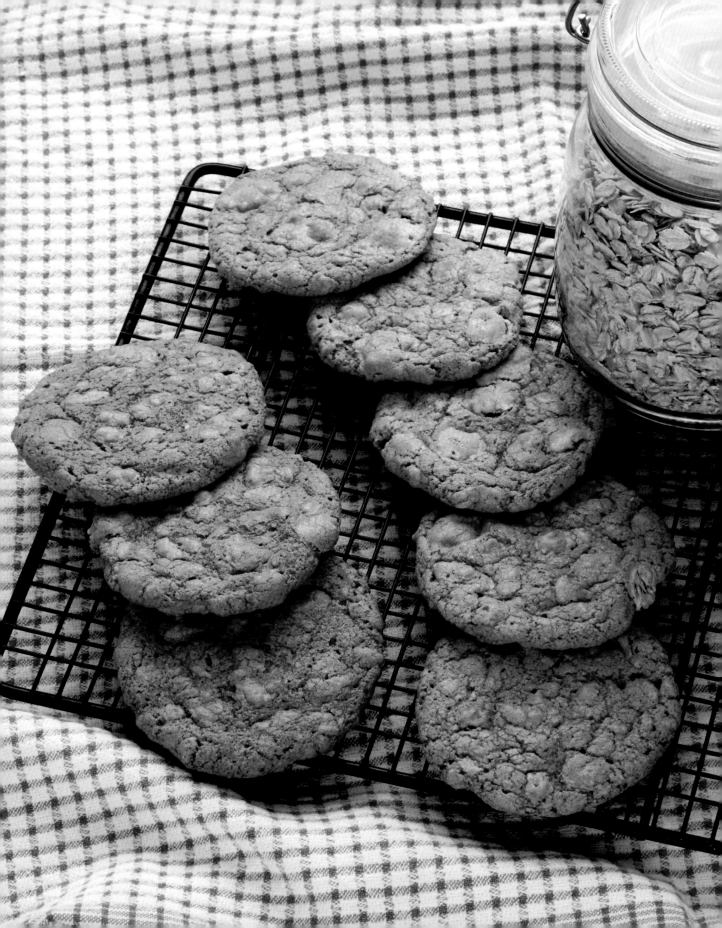

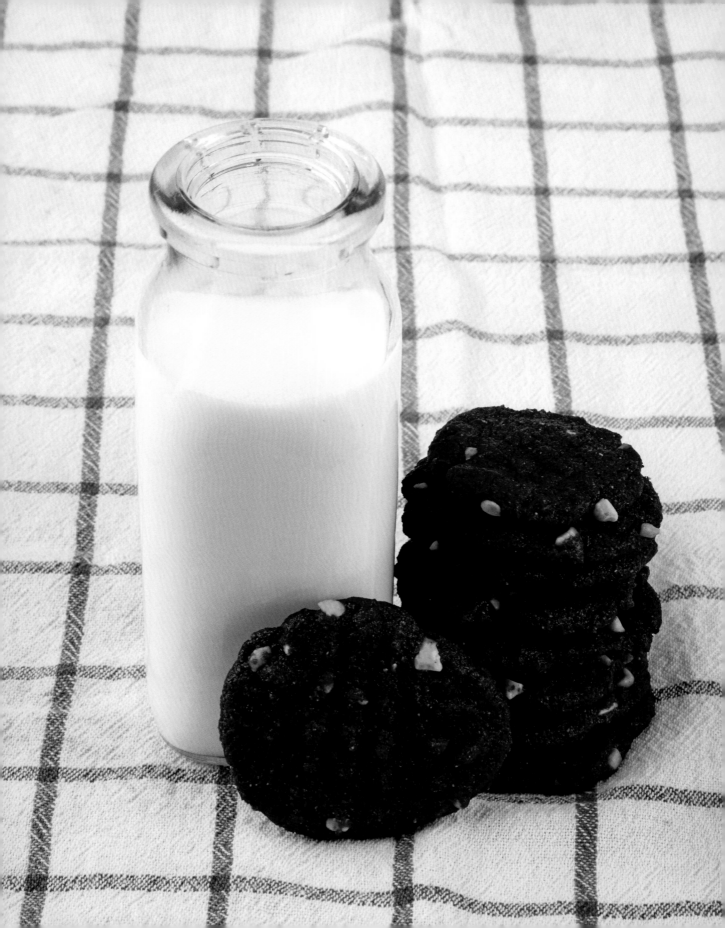

Peanut Butter Cocoa Snaps VEG · *Makes 62 (2-inch) cookies*

AFTER TWO MARRIAGES AND ONE STILL ON THE BOOKS, I finally learned that the key to a lasting relationship is a combination of habits, lifestyles, likes, a sense of humour, outlooks, respect, and beliefs that complement each other. What does this have to do with a cookie? Well, a perfect cookie is all about the right combinations too. Without the perfect mix of flavours and textures, a cookie, just like a marriage, can be a total bust.

½ cup canola oil (see page 183)

½ cup natural peanut butter, smooth or crunchy

1¼ cups packed dark brown sugar

1 omega-3 egg

½ cup natural cocoa powder

2 tsp pure vanilla extract

1 cup whole grain barley flour

½ tsp baking soda

1. Place a rack in the middle of the oven and preheat the oven to 350°F. Line a rimless baking sheet with parchment paper.

2. In a medium bowl, using a hand-held electric mixer, beat together the oil and peanut butter. Add the brown sugar, egg, and cocoa powder and beat on low speed until thick and creamy, 2 to 3 minutes. Add 1 Tbsp water and the vanilla and beat until blended.

3. Add the flour and baking soda and gently beat until combined.

4. Using a 1-teaspoon ice-cream scoop with a release button, measure out and drop the dough onto the prepared pan. You should be able to fit 15 cookies on the baking sheet. Using a fork, gently press down to flatten the tops of the cookies and leave a fork imprint. Slide the fork out and then, at a 90-degree angle, press the fork down to complete the basket-weave pattern. If the fork starts sticking to the dough, wipe with a paper towel before continuing.

5. Bake the cookies for 10 to 11 minutes until the tops are dry, then remove from the oven and let sit on the baking sheet for 2 minutes. Transfer the cookies to a wire cooling rack and let them cool completely, or they will fall apart when you eat them. Finish baking the rest of the dough.

6. Store the cookies in a covered container for up to 1 week or freeze for up to 3 months.

1 SERVING = 2 COOKIES
PER SERVING: 113 CALORIES, 6.1 G TOTAL FAT, 0.7 G SATURATED FAT, 0 G TRANS FAT, 6 MG CHOLESTEROL, 22 MG SODIUM, 13.9 G CARBOHYDRATE, 1.5 G FIBRE, 9.3 G SUGARS, 9 G ADDED SUGARS, 1.8 G PROTEIN, 79 MG POTASSIUM
CARBOHYDRATE CHOICE = 1 CHOICE

Spicy Ginger Molasses Cookies VEG · *Makes 46 (3-inch) cookies*

THIS COOKIE WAS INSPIRED BY THE WINNING RECIPE in a *Cityline* Christmas cookie contest. It was truly excellent, but because I can't leave well enough alone and I wanted them to be higher in fibre and lower in saturated fat, I tweaked them—not to be confused with twerking—and voilà! These are perfect for a cookie party or a cookie exchange.

2¾ cups whole grain barley flour

2 tsp ground ginger

1 tsp ground cinnamon

½ tsp ground cloves

1 tsp baking soda

¼ cup unsalted butter, room temperature

½ cup canola oil (see page 183)

1 cup granulated sugar

1 omega-3 egg

¼ cup molasses

½ cup diced dried candied ginger (see note)

¼ cup turbinado sugar or coarse or sanding sugar (see page 184)

1 SERVING = 1 COOKIE
PER SERVING: 95 CALORIES, 3.7 G TOTAL FAT, 0.9 G SATURATED FAT, 0 G TRANS FAT, 7 MG CHOLESTEROL, 31 MG SODIUM, 14.7 G CARBOHYDRATE, 1.2 G FIBRE, 8.8 G SUGARS, 8.7 G ADDED SUGARS, 0.9 G PROTEIN, 87 MG POTASSIUM
CARBOHYDRATE CHOICE = 1 CHOICE

1. Place a rack in the middle of the oven and preheat the oven to 350°F. Line a rimless baking sheet with parchment paper. Set aside.

2. In a medium bowl, whisk together the flour, ground ginger, cinnamon, cloves, and baking soda. Set aside.

3. In a large bowl, using a hand-held electric mixer, cream the butter. Add the canola oil and granulated sugar and beat until the batter turns light and fluffy. Add the egg and beat well. Add 1 Tbsp water and the molasses and beat in.

4. Add the flour mixture and mix in on low speed. Add the candied ginger and stir well.

5. Using a 1-tablespoon ice-cream scoop with a release button, scoop out the cookie dough and, using your hands, roll into 1-inch balls. Spread the turbinado or coarse sugar out on a shallow plate, and gently press the top of each cookie ball into the sugar to coat. Place the cookie balls, sugar side up, on the baking sheet about 2 inches apart. You will get about 9 cookies per sheet. Gently press the tops down.

6. Bake in the oven for 15 to 18 minutes, until the tops crack and the cookies are golden.

7. Rest the cookies on the baking sheet for 3 minutes, then transfer to a wire rack to cool completely. Repeat with the remaining dough.

8. Store the cookies in a covered container for up to 1 week or freeze for up to 3 months.

NOTE: There are three styles of candied ginger. One style comes in a jar in a heavy sugar syrup. Another is sold in small cubes, which you would add to a Christmas cake recipe. The most common style, and the type I use in my recipes, is sold in small, thin pieces and is labelled "dried ginger slices" or "crystalized ginger" or "dried candied ginger." This type of ginger has been sliced, cooked in a sugar syrup, coated with sugar, and allowed to dry. You can find it in the baking section of a large grocery store.

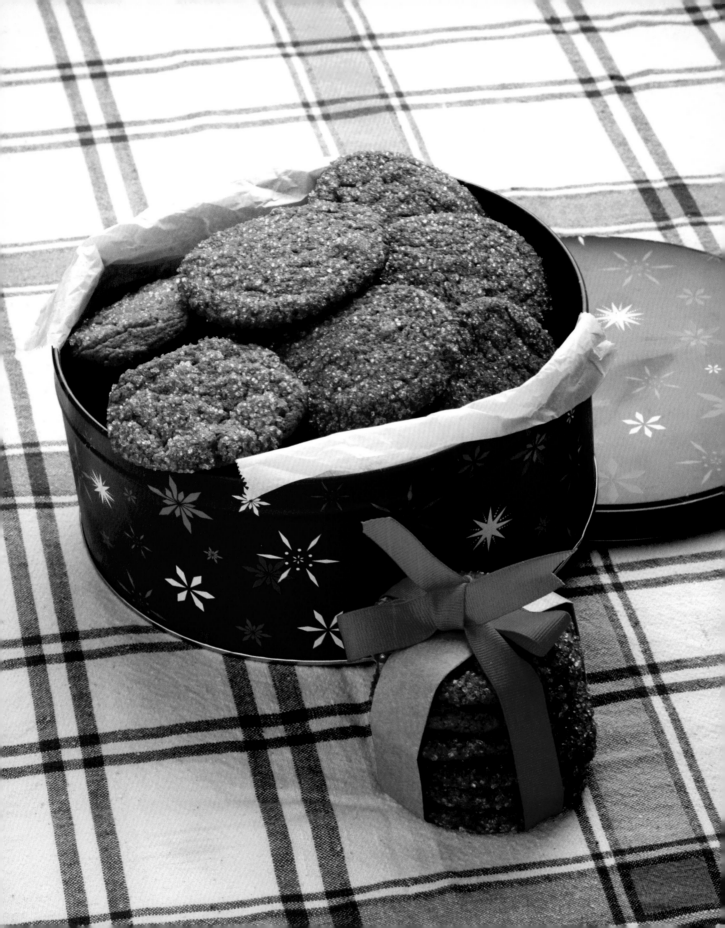

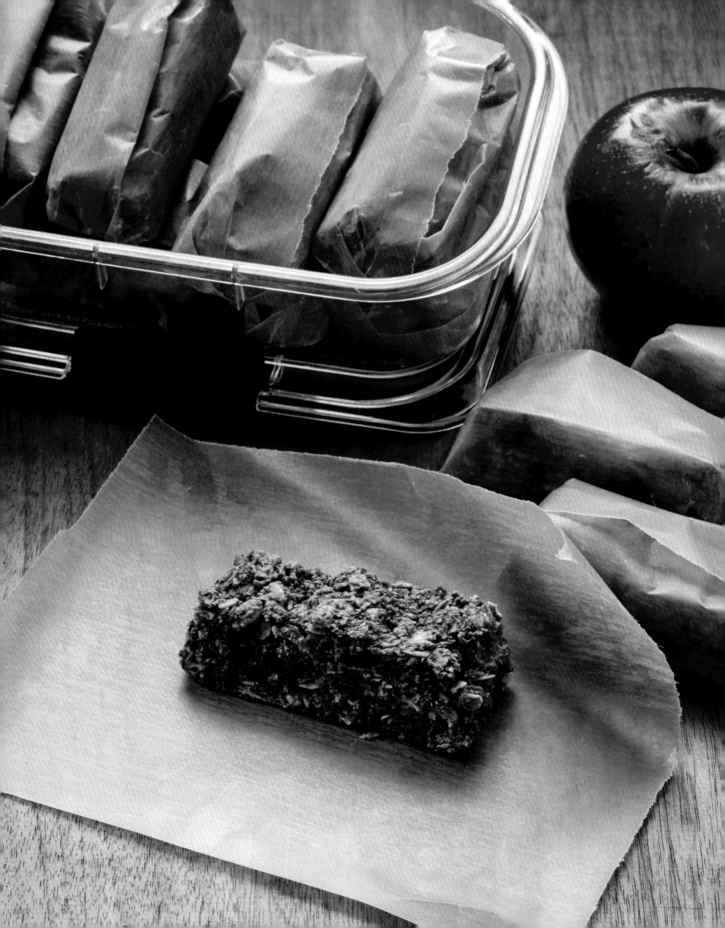

Snack Bars   VEG · *Makes 24 bars*

IT'S 4 P.M. AND YOU'RE HUNGRY, CRABBY, AND ANGRY. If someone even dares to look at you the wrong way, having a full-blown tantrum seems like a normal option. You're hangry. These nut-free snack bars are loaded with soluble fibre, which will help fill you up no matter what time of day you eat them. Just remember that as you increase your fibre intake, you need to increase your fluid intake, or you and your digestive system will be hangry at each other.

2 cups large oat flakes

1½ cups oat bran

1 cup whole grain barley flour

1½ cups ground flaxseed
(see page 184)

1 cup dark or bittersweet
chocolate chips

1½ cups whole pitted dates

½ cup canola oil (see page 183)

2 omega-3 eggs

1 cup packed dark brown sugar

2 Tbsp natural cocoa powder

2 Tbsp ground cinnamon

1 Tbsp pure vanilla extract

NOTE: Kids don't need as much fibre as adults, so cut the bars into 48 squares if you are making these for children under 12. See the chart on page 4.

1. Place a rack in the middle of the oven and preheat the oven to 375°F. Line a 9 × 13-inch baking pan with wet parchment paper (see page 15), wringing it out well and making sure that there is some overhang so you can pick up the cooked snack bars.

2. In a large bowl, mix together the dry ingredients: oat flakes, oat bran, flour, flaxseed, and chocolate chips.

3. In the bowl of a food processor fitted with the steel blade attachment, pulse the dates, oil, ¼ cup water, eggs, sugar, cocoa, cinnamon, and vanilla. It will be noisy and, depending on how old your food processor is, it might dance around on the counter. Purée until there are only small specks of dates visible.

4. Transfer the date mixture to the dry ingredients, using a rubber spatula to get as much out of the food processor as you can. Using a large wooden spoon, stir until well combined and there are no visible signs of dry flour. I always end up using my hands.

5. The batter will be sticky, so just plop it into the prepared pan and spread it out. Then, lightly dampen your hands and press the mixture down so that it's evenly spread out. You can also use the back of a spoon for this.

6. Bake for 25 to 27 minutes, until the top is a deep golden brown. Remove from the oven and let cool in the pan for 5 minutes to set.

7. Using the excess parchment paper on the sides, lift the bar out of the pan and place on a wire rack to cool completely, parchment paper and all. Cut into 24 bars. Store in an airtight container for up to 2 weeks or freeze for up to 3 months. I like to wrap them up in waxed paper and then freeze them in bags. On a day when I think I might get stuck somewhere around the witching hour— a.k.a. 4 p.m.—I'll pop one into my bag and know I've got a healthy snack ready and waiting and calling my name.

1 SERVING = 1 BAR
PER SERVING: 272 CALORIES, 12.5 G TOTAL FAT, 2.7 G SATURATED FAT, 0 G TRANS FAT, 16 MG CHOLESTEROL, 12 MG SODIUM, 39.6 G CARBOHYDRATE, 6.3 G FIBRE, 19.4 G SUGARS, 15.1 G ADDED SUGARS, 5.7 G PROTEIN, 279 MG POTASSIUM
CARBOHYDRATE CHOICE = 2 CHOICES

My Mom's Matrimonial Squares   VEG · *Makes 16 squares*

WHEN MY SIBLINGS AND I STARTED CLEANING OUT my parents' home of 30 years, we were overwhelmed, to say the very least. My parents had a lot of stuff. They'd been raised during the Depression and their mindset had always been that you never knew when you'd need . . . (fill in the blank). When we were sorting through their treasures, I was lucky enough to score my mom's cookbooks, which included her recipe for matrimonial cake. The ingredients were clearly written in mom's handwriting, but the method was cryptic: "Cook to a smooth paste then add lemon. Cool. 350° till brown." I spent a nostalgic afternoon going through her cookbooks and recipe files, and my childhood appeared before me via the food she loved to cook for us. In honour of my mom, here is my version of one of her go-to desserts.

FILLING

1 medium Cara Cara or regular navel orange (see note)

2 cups whole pitted dates

1 tsp pure vanilla extract

BASE

2½ cups large oat flakes (divided)

1 cup whole walnuts

½ cup flaxseed meal (see page 184)

½ cup packed dark brown sugar

¼ cup unsalted butter

¼ cup canola oil (see page 183)

1. Make the filling. Rinse and dry the orange. Zest the orange and set the zest aside. Cut off the remaining peel and then cut the orange into small ½-inch pieces.

2. Pour 1 cup water into a small saucepan and heat on high until boiling. Add the dates and orange pieces and bring back to a boil. Cover, reduce heat to low, and simmer until the dates start to soften, about 2 minutes, depending on how hard they were. Remove the lid and continue to simmer, uncovered, until the dates and orange pieces become a paste, about 5 minutes. Stir frequently. You don't want to see anything that looks like a date. When it's ready, remove from heat, add the vanilla and orange zest, and set aside to cool.

3. Place a rack in the middle of the oven and preheat the oven to 350°F. Line an 8-inch square baking pan with wet parchment paper (see page 15). Wring it out well, making sure there is some overhang so you can pick up the cooked squares. Pat the inside of the lined pan with a paper towel to absorb any extra water.

4. Make the base. Pour 2 cups oat flakes into the bowl of a food processor fitted with the steel blade attachment and pulse until it looks like a coarse flour. Transfer the ground oat flakes to a large bowl. Add the walnuts to the food processor and pulse until they are finely ground, then add the ground oats. Add the flaxseed meal, the remaining ½ cup oat flakes, and the brown sugar to the oat mixture and stir together using a fork, making sure that the brown sugar is well distributed.

5. Melt the butter in a microwave-safe bowl, then add the oil and stir well. Pour into the oat mixture and stir until it looks like wet sand. Tip half of this mixture into the prepared pan and press down firmly to make a crust (take your time here, otherwise the crust will fall apart when you cut it).

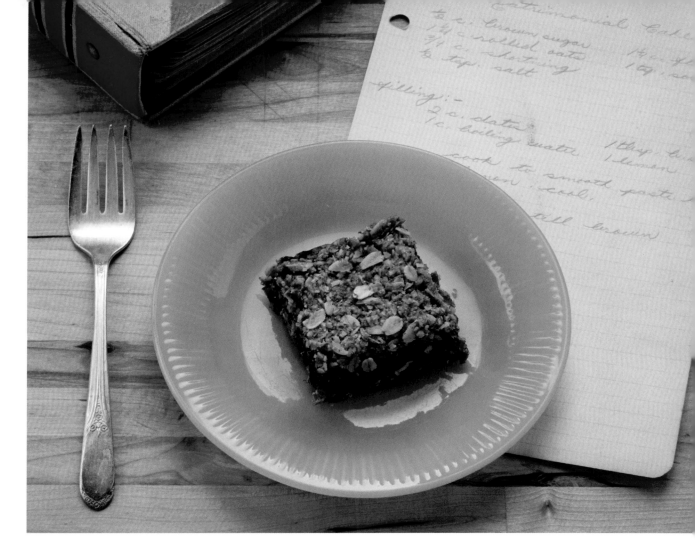

NOTE: A Cara Cara orange is a red-fleshed navel orange that is sweeter than your average navel orange, making it perfect for this recipe. I like to try and reduce as much of the added sugars as possible without sacrificing flavour and texture in all my baking. If you can't find a Cara Cara orange, use a regular navel orange.

6. Spoon the date mixture on top of the oat mixture in the pan, spreading it out evenly. Sprinkle the remaining oat mixture over top and lightly press down.

7. Bake for 22 to 25 minutes, until the edges are golden brown. Cool the pan on a wire rack for 10 minutes.

8. Using the excess parchment paper, lift the square out of the pan and place on the wire rack, parchment paper and all. Let cool completely, then cut into 16 equal portions. Store any leftovers in an airtight container for up to 4 days.

1 SERVING = 1 SQUARE
PER SERVING: 270 CALORIES, 13.4 G TOTAL FAT, 2.8 G SATURATED FAT, 0 G TRANS FAT, 8 MG CHOLESTEROL, 5 MG SODIUM, 36.4 G CARBOHYDRATE, 4.9 G FIBRE, 20.4 G SUGARS, 7.1 G ADDED SUGARS, 4.7 G PROTEIN, 268 MG POTASSIUM
CARBOHYDRATE CHOICE = 2 CHOICES

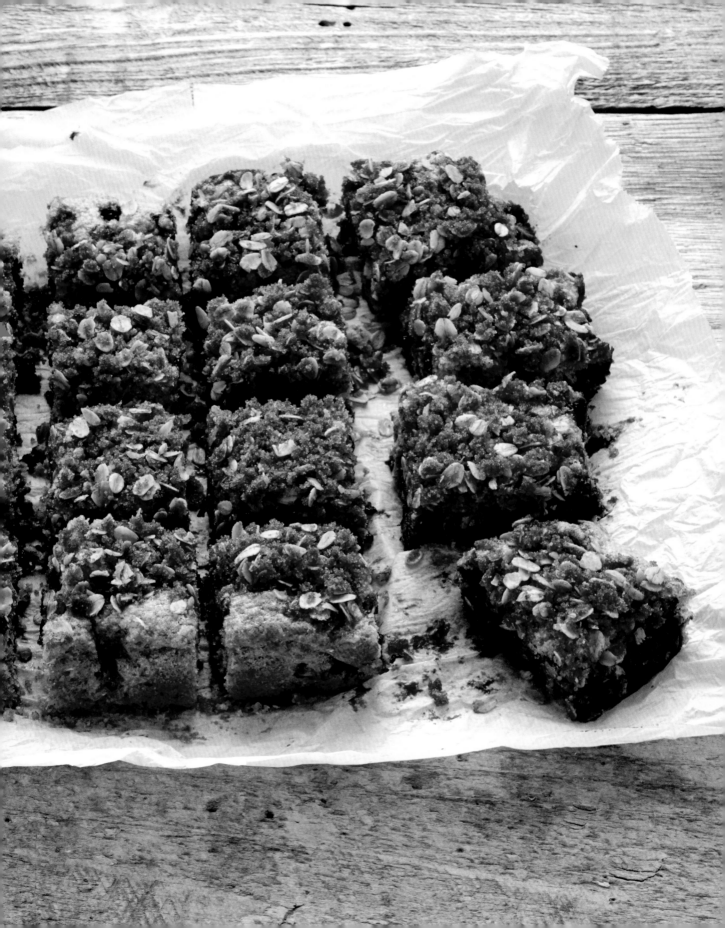

Blueberry Buckle   VEG · *Makes 16 squares*

I ONCE MADE THIS DESSERT FOR OUR WONDERFUL FRIENDS, Jill and Larry, my husband, and my son, Andrew. Jill, my husband, and I ate our one serving like normal dessert-eating people would, and Larry and Andrew ate all but one piece. And as we waved goodbye to Jill and Larry, Larry got out of his car, came back into the house, and ate the last piece. It's that good.

3 cups fresh (not frozen) local blueberries

TOPPING

½ cup packed dark brown sugar

½ cup large oat flakes

1 tsp ground cinnamon

2 Tbsp canola oil (see page 183)

BUCKLE

1½ cups whole grain barley flour

½ cup medium-grind cornmeal (see note on page 74)

2 Tbsp flaxseed meal (see page 184)

2 tsp baking powder

½ cup skim milk

¼ cup unsalted butter, room temperature

¼ cup canola oil (see page 183)

½ cup granulated sugar

2 omega-3 eggs

1 tsp pure vanilla extract

1. Place a rack in the middle of the oven and preheat the oven to 350°F. Line a 9-inch square baking pan with wet parchment paper (see page 15), shake out any excess water, pat dry, and set aside.

2. Pick through the blueberries for stems and discard. Rinse well in a strainer. Shake out water and lay the blueberries on a clean tea towel or paper towel to air-dry.

3. Make the topping. In a small bowl, mix together the brown sugar, oat flakes, cinnamon, and oil. Set aside.

4. Make the buckle. In a medium bowl, whisk together the flour, cornmeal, flaxseed meal, and baking powder. Set aside.

5. Measure out the milk and have it ready to go.

6. In a large bowl, using a hand-held electric mixer, beat the butter until soft and fluffy. Add the oil and gently beat in. Add the sugar and beat in. Add the eggs one at a time, beating after each addition until the mixture is a light lemon-yellow. Beat in the vanilla.

7. Add half of the flour mixture, beating very gently until there is no flour visible. Pour in all the milk at once and gently beat in.

8. Add the rest of the flour mixture and gently beat in. Remove the beaters and scrape off as much of the batter as possible.

9. Check on the blueberries, and if they are still wet, pat them dry. Gently fold the berries into the cake batter.

10. Scrape the batter out into the prepared pan and smooth out the top. Evenly sprinkle the topping over top. Bake for 45 to 50 minutes or until a cake tester inserted into the middle of the cake comes out clean.

recipe continues

1 SERVING = 1 SQUARE
PER SERVING: 228 CALORIES, 12.7 G TOTAL
FAT, 4.4 G SATURATED FAT, 0 G TRANS FAT,
40 MG CHOLESTEROL, 64 MG SODIUM,
33 G CARBOHYDRATE, 3.6 G FIBRE,
17.2 G SUGARS, 13.7 G ADDED SUGARS,
3.3 G PROTEIN, 119 MG POTASSIUM
CARBOHYDRATE CHOICE = 2 CHOICES

11. Remove the buckle from the oven and let cool in the pan
    for 5 minutes. After 5 minutes, remove the buckle from
    the pan by pulling on the parchment paper edges and
    set it on a wire rack to cool. If you forget to remove it
    from the pan, the buckle will steam and become wet.
    When it is cool enough to handle, cut into 16 equal
    pieces and serve slightly warm or at room temperature.
    Store any leftovers in an airtight container for up to 2 days.

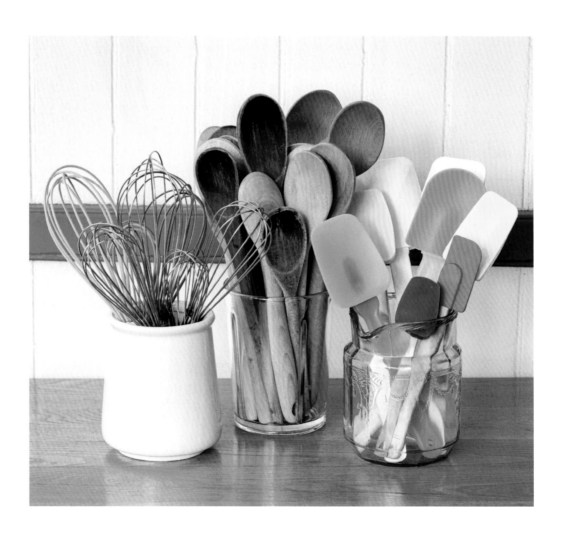

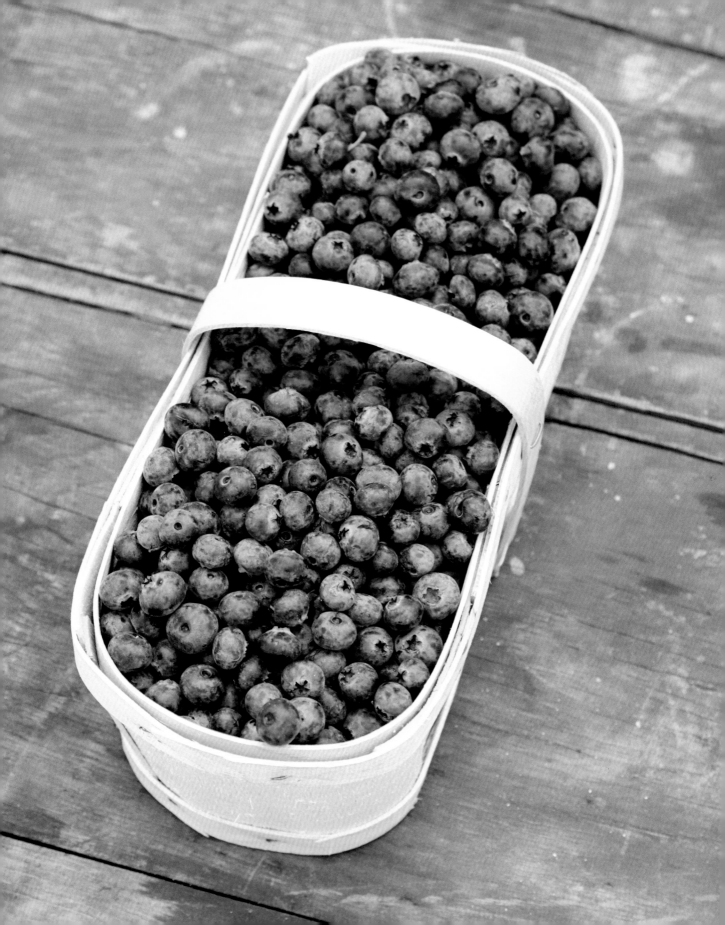

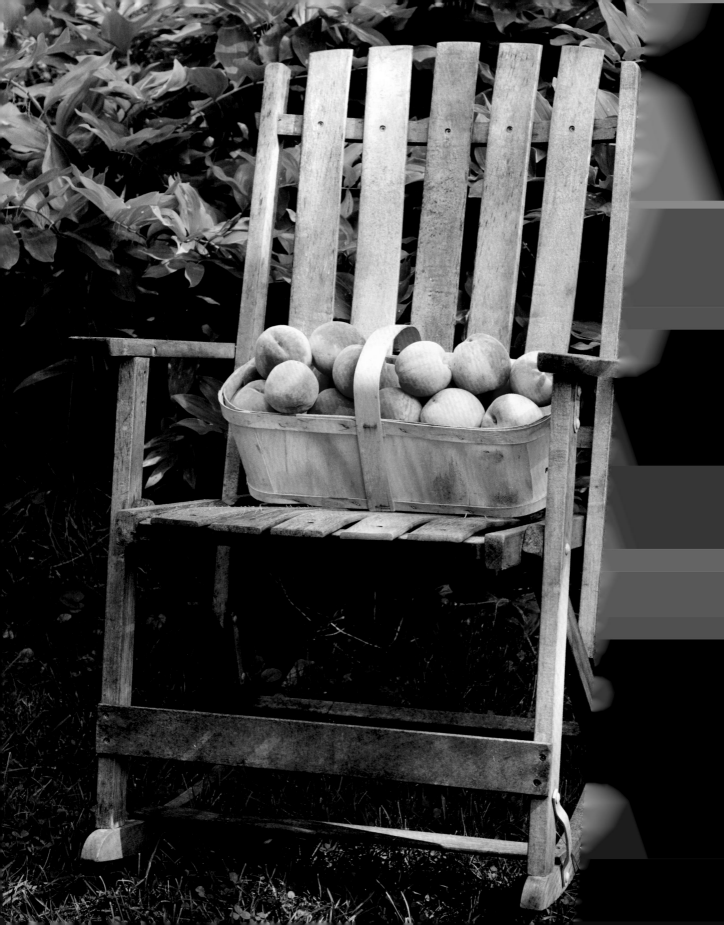

Peach & Blueberry Galette   VEG · *Serves 8*

SOME PEOPLE ARE INSPIRED BY MUSIC, others are inspired by art, and I'm inspired by food. Show me a bowl of fresh, ripe peaches and I can come up with at least 10 delicious things to make with them—throw in some fresh blueberries and the number doubles. This recipe was inspired by ripe peaches on my counter, blueberries in my fridge, and the question, "What should I make for dessert?" Galettes are rustic-looking open-faced pies stuffed with seasonal fruits and berries. They're so much easier to bake than a pie, you'll be making this all peach season.

GALETTE PASTRY

1½ cups whole grain barley flour, plus extra for rolling pastry

¼ cup flaxseed meal
(see page 184)

1 Tbsp granulated sugar

½ cup cold unsalted butter, cut in 1-inch cubes

3 Tbsp ice-cold water

FILLING

3 cups peeled peaches, cut in 1-inch slices (3 to 6 medium peaches)

1¼ cups fresh (not frozen) local blueberries, rinsed and patted dry

½ cup packed dark brown sugar

1 Tbsp + 1 tsp minute tapioca (see note on page 212)

1 tsp ground cinnamon

TOPPING

1 Tbsp orange zest

1 Tbsp coarse or sanding sugar

1 tsp skim milk

Ice cream, for serving (optional)

1. Make the pastry. In a food processor fitted with the steel blade attachment, pulse together the flour, flaxseed meal, and sugar. Add the butter and pulse until it becomes the size of small peas. Turn the food processor on and add the ice-cold water through the feed tube. Let the dough come together; if it appears too dry, add an extra tablespoon of ice water.

2. Remove the dough from the processor, place on some plastic wrap, and shape into a 6-inch disc. Refrigerate for at least 30 minutes and up to 2 days.

3. When you want to start the galette, make sure the rack is in the middle of the oven and preheat the oven to 400°F. Have a large rimmed baking sheet ready.

4. Take the pastry out of the fridge. Let it warm up slightly as you prepare the filling.

5. To make the filling, gently combine the sliced peaches, blueberries, sugar, tapioca, and cinnamon. Set aside.

6. Place an 18-inch piece of parchment paper on your counter. Sprinkle 1 tsp barley flour onto the parchment paper, remove the pastry disc from the plastic wrap, and place the pastry in the middle of the parchment paper. Lightly dust the top with a teeny bit of flour, then roll out the pastry into a 12-inch circle. I use a silicone rolling pin for this, and easy does it here, as this pastry is very tender. Keep rolling gently until the pastry is about ⅛ inch thick. Pick up the parchment paper with the pastry and place onto the baking sheet.

7. Carefully tip the filling into the centre of the pastry, leaving a 2-inch border. It's okay to have the fruit slightly mounded in the middle.

recipe continues

1 SERVING = ⅛ OF THE GALETTE WITHOUT ICE CREAM
PER SERVING: 340 CALORIES, 14.6 TOTAL FAT, 7.5 G SATURATED FAT, 0 G TRANS FAT, 31 MG CHOLESTEROL, 10 MG SODIUM, 46.6 G CARBOHYDRATE, 6.8 G FIBRE, 25 G SUGARS, 17.3 ADDED SUGARS, 3.8 G PROTEIN, 256 MG POTASSIUM
CARBOHYDRATE CHOICE = 2½ CHOICES

8. Fold the border of the pastry up and over top of the fruit, forming a rough edge. Continue around the entire galette, being careful not to tear the pastry.

9. Mix the orange zest with the sugar. Using a pastry brush or your fingers, brush the milk onto the pastry, then sprinkle the orange sugar on top, pressing the sugar into the pastry.

10. Bake for 30 to 35 minutes, until the pastry is golden brown. Remove the galette from the oven and place on a wire rack to cool. When completely cooled, cut into eight wedges and serve with or without ice cream.

NOTE: Tapioca is a type of thickener that is often used in pies and crisps. Find it in the grocery store where they sell cornstarch.

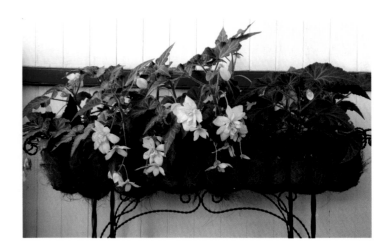

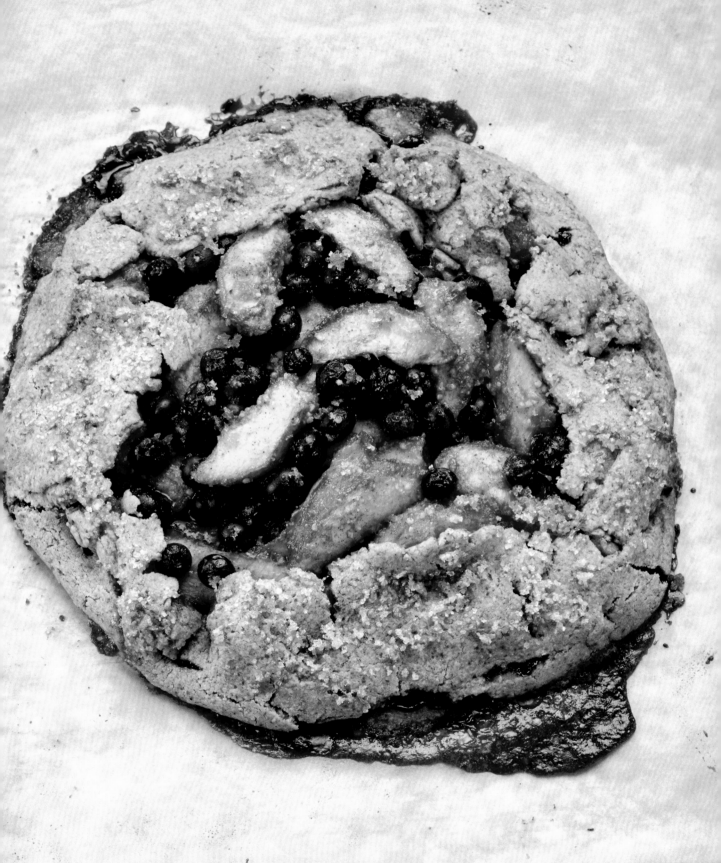

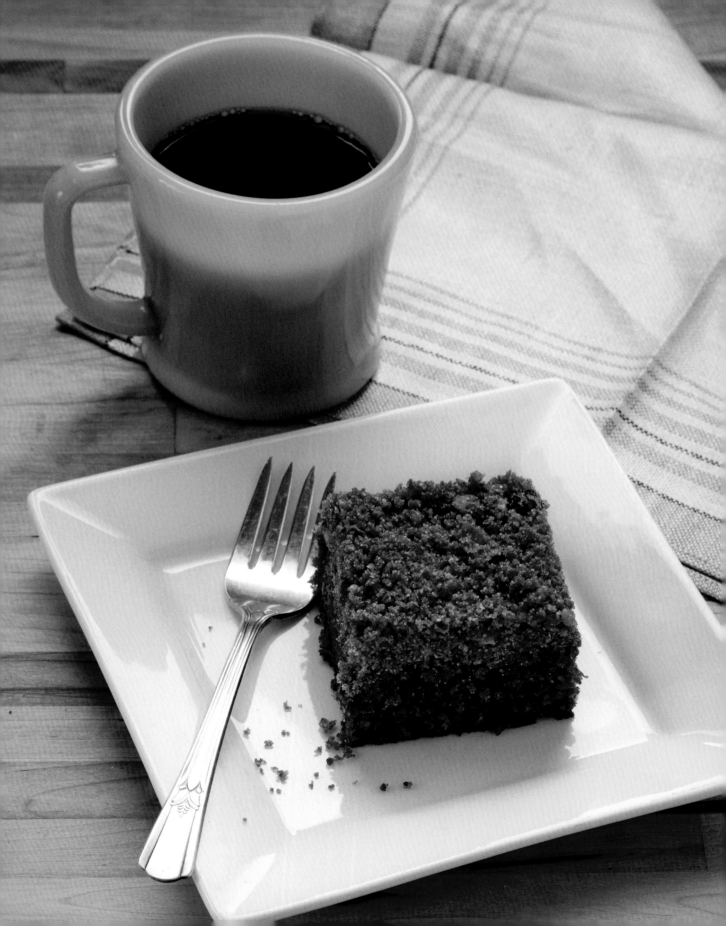

Pumpkin Spice Crumble Coffee Cake VEG · *Makes 16 squares*

EVEN THOUGH I LOVE THE TASTE OF PUMPKIN, I'm not a huge fan of pumpkin pie. I don't love the texture of custard, and moreover, pumpkin pie wasn't a tradition at our house on Thanksgiving. My brother and grandpa had birthdays around that time, so we always had birthday cake instead and said, "we are thankful for our lives, and happy birthday, John and Gramps." Here's my spin on pumpkin pie, minus the pastry, whipped cream, and filling—which basically makes it a cake.

TOPPING

½ cup packed dark brown sugar

¾ cup whole grain barley flour

1 tsp ground cinnamon

½ cup whole pecans, chopped

½ cup diced dried candied ginger (see note on page 200)

¼ cup canola oil (see page 183)

COFFEE CAKE

⅓ cup canola oil (see page 183)

¾ cup packed dark brown sugar

2 omega-3 eggs

1 cup pure pumpkin purée (see note on page 41)

1 tsp pure vanilla extract

¾ cup 1% buttermilk (see note)

1 cup oat bran

1 cup whole grain barley flour

1 tsp baking powder

1 tsp baking soda

1 Tbsp ground cinnamon

½ tsp ground ginger

⅛ tsp ground cloves

⅛ tsp ground allspice

NOTE: To make this lactose-free, substitute either original almond or soy beverage plus 1 Tbsp apple cider vinegar for the buttermilk.

1. Place a rack in the middle of the oven and preheat the oven to 350°F. Line a 9-inch square pan with wet parchment paper (see page 15). Make sure there is some overhang so you can lift the cake out later.

2. Make the topping. In a medium bowl, mix together the brown sugar, flour, cinnamon, pecans, and candied ginger. Pour in the oil and mix until the topping looks wet and crumbly. Set aside.

3. Make the cake. In a large bowl, whisk together the oil, brown sugar, eggs, pumpkin purée, vanilla, and buttermilk until well blended. Add the oat bran and whisk until it is well combined. Set aside for 10 minutes. The oat bran is going to absorb some of the liquid. Don't scrimp on this rest time or the cake will be wet.

4. While you are waiting, whisk together the flour, baking powder, baking soda, cinnamon, ginger, cloves, and allspice in a small bowl.

5. Transfer the dry ingredients to the oat bran mixture and beat in using the whisk. Beat for at least 1 minute and no more than 2 minutes. This will develop the gluten in the barley flour, which traps air bubbles and helps the cake to rise.

6. Pour into the prepared pan, spreading out the batter evenly. Evenly sprinkle the topping over top and then place into the oven.

7. Bake for 40 to 45 minutes or until a toothpick inserted in the middle of the cake comes out clean. Let cool on a wire rack for 10 minutes and then, using the excess parchment paper on the sides, lift the cake out of the pan and place on the wire rack to cool completely, parchment paper and all. Cut into 16 equal pieces and serve. Store any leftovers in an airtight container for up to 2 days.

1 SERVING = 1 SQUARE
PER SERVING: 267 CALORIES, 11.8 G TOTAL FAT, 0.9 G SATURATED FAT, 0 G TRANS FAT, 25 MG CHOLESTEROL, 142 MG SODIUM, 36.1 G CARBOHYDRATE, 3.7 G FIBRE, 24.5 G SUGARS, 21.8 G ADDED SUGARS, 4.1 G PROTEIN, 258 MG POTASSIUM
CARBOHYDRATE CHOICE = 2 CHOICES

Rhubarb Crumble with Strawberries & Ginger VEG LF · *Serves 10*

MOTHER NATURE IS PART WONDER, PART MAGIC, AND PART SCIENCE. She's unpredictable and altogether her own boss, which makes for an interesting combo. Depending on her weather whim, local rhubarb and strawberries are either available at the same time, or they just aren't. I've learned that she can't be trusted, so I've got my bases covered when it comes to this recipe: when the rhubarb comes up, I freeze enough to make this dessert so I'm ready when the local strawberries hit the market.

CRISP

5 cups chopped rhubarb, cut in 1-inch pieces

3 cups strawberries, rinsed, tops removed, and halved

¼ cup liquid honey

1 Tbsp minute tapioca (see note on page 212)

1 tsp grated fresh ginger

TOPPING

1 cup large oat flakes

⅓ cup whole grain barley flour or whole grain oat flour

½ cup oat bran

¼ cup natural wheat germ

2 Tbsp flaxseed meal (see page 184)

½ cup packed dark brown sugar

¼ cup + 2 Tbsp finely diced dried candied ginger (see note on page 200)

1 Tbsp ground cinnamon

½ cup canola oil (see page 183)

1. Place a rack in the middle of the oven and preheat the oven to 350°F. Line an 8 × 11-inch glass or ceramic casserole dish with wet parchment paper (see page 15). Set aside.

2. Make the crisp. In a large bowl, mix together the rhubarb, strawberries, honey, tapioca, and ginger. Transfer to the prepared dish.

3. Make the topping. In a medium bowl, stir together the oat flakes, flour, oat bran, wheat germ, flaxseed meal, brown sugar, candied ginger, and cinnamon. Add the oil and mix with a fork until well combined. The mixture should look wet. Spread the topping evenly over the rhubarb and strawberries.

4. Bake for 45 to 50 minutes, until the topping is golden brown and the rhubarb is soft. Let sit for at least 30 minutes before serving. Serve warm or cold. This will keep for up to 2 days in the fridge.

NOTE: Honey should never be given to a child under the age of 12 months. According to Health Canada, "Infant botulism is caused by *Clostridium botulinum* spores, which are sometimes found in both pasteurized and unpasteurized honey. When an infant ingests honey, bacteria from these spores can grow and produce toxins that could lead to paralysis."

1 SERVING = ¹⁄₁₀ OF THE CRUMBLE
PER SERVING: 313 CALORIES, 13.7 G TOTAL FAT, 1.2 G SATURATED FAT, 0 G TRANS FAT, 0 MG CHOLESTEROL, 8 MG SODIUM, 48.3 G CARBOHYDRATE, 5.6 G FIBRE, 26.6 G SUGARS, 23.5 G ADDED SUGARS, 4.8 G PROTEIN, 493 MG POTASSIUM
CARBOHYDRATE CHOICE = 3 CHOICES

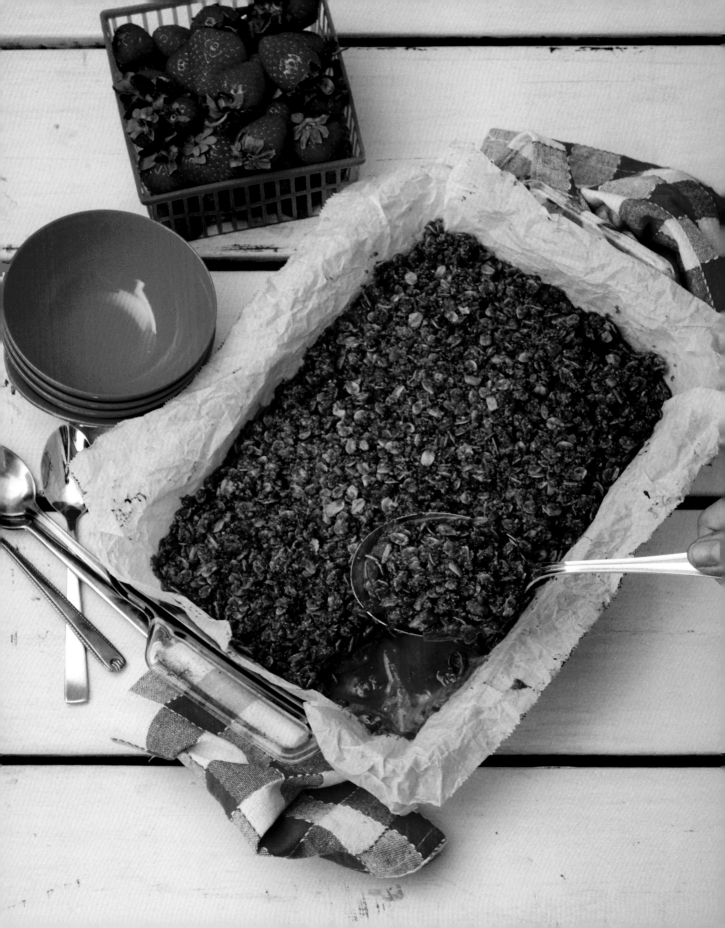

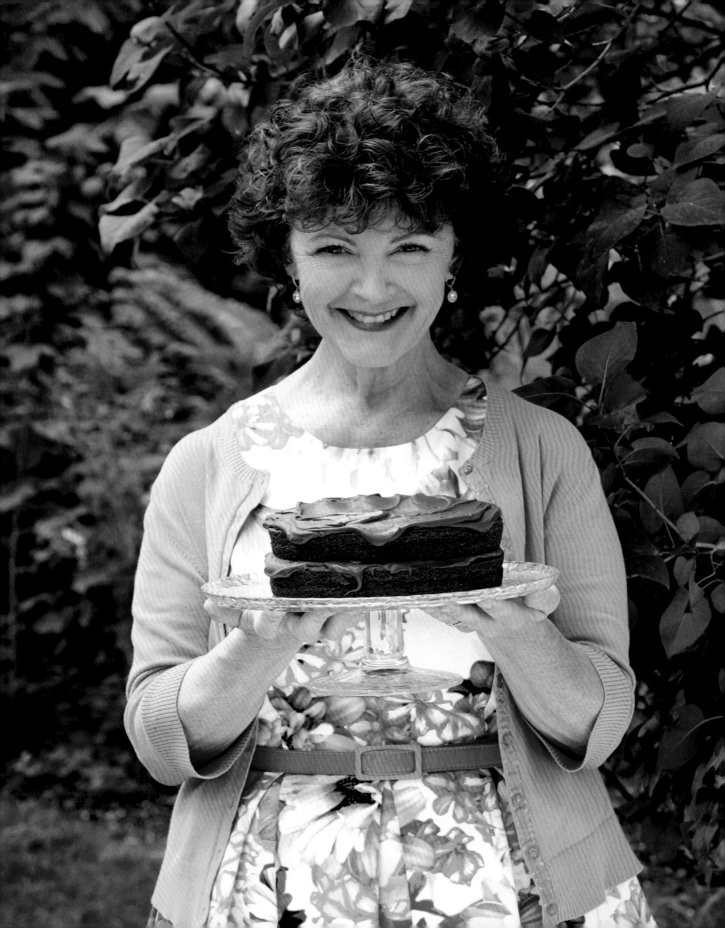

Chocolate Fudge Cake   VEG · *Serves 16*

NECESSITY HAS OFTEN BEEN CALLED THE MOTHER OF INVENTION. It was also called some other interesting metaphors the day I found out that baby-food stewed prunes were too hard to find in most grocery stores. The situation was made much worse because I had a craving for my go-to signature chocolate cake. I decided to make my own stewed prunes, but with a professional home economist spin, in a food processor. Thank you, Necessity—you spearheaded another brilliant recipe.

1 cup whole pitted prunes

¾ cup natural cocoa powder

1 cup granulated sugar

1 cup chocolate soy beverage

¼ cup canola oil (see page 183)

1 Tbsp pure vanilla extract

2 tsp apple cider vinegar

1 omega-3 egg

1½ cups whole grain spelt flour or whole wheat flour (see note)

1½ tsp baking soda

ICING

¼ cup unsalted butter or non-hydrogenated margarine

¼ cup chocolate soy beverage

1½ cups icing sugar, sifted

½ cup natural cocoa powder, sifted

1 tsp pure vanilla extract

NOTE: If you can't find whole grain spelt flour, feel free to use whole wheat flour. Whole wheat flour is not a whole grain because the germ has been removed, unless it is stone-milled whole wheat flour.

1. Place the prunes and 1 cup water into a small saucepan. Bring to a boil, cover, then remove from heat and let sit for at least 15 minutes and up to 1 hour. When cool, proceed.

2. Place a rack in the middle of the oven and preheat the oven to 350°F. Lightly spray two 8-inch round cake pans with oil and either sprinkle gently with flour or line the bottoms with parchment paper. Set aside.

3. Sift the cocoa powder onto a piece of wax paper or into a bowl, and set aside.

4. Pour the prunes into the bowl of a food processor fitted with the steel blade attachment. Add the cocoa powder and pulse until combined and smooth.

5. Add the sugar, chocolate soy beverage, oil, vanilla, vinegar, and egg to the food processor. Process until smooth.

6. Add the flour to the food processor and pulse until combined. Continue to process for at least 1 minute; the batter shouldn't be lumpy. Add the baking soda and pulse for 20 seconds (the baking soda will start reacting to the vinegar right away and the batter will start swelling). Quickly divide the batter equally between the two pans. Lightly spread out the top of the batter so it's even.

7. Bake the cakes for 25 to 30 minutes or until a toothpick inserted in the centre of the cakes comes out clean.

8. Cool on a wire rack for 10 minutes, then remove the cakes from the pans and continue cooling on the wire rack.

9. Make the icing. Put the butter or margarine and chocolate

recipe continues

NOTE: The only other person in the entire world who has made my "Don't Forget to Leave Room for Chocolate Cake" more than I have is my friend and fellow professional home economist Jennifer Dyck. She recipe-tested this version and served it for Canada's 150th birthday to her extended family, and it got raves from both young and old. It's another chocolate cake winner.

NOTE: If you use non-hydrogenated margarine for the icing, this cake is lactose-free.

soy beverage in a microwave-safe dish. Heat on medium for 45 seconds. Whisk until the butter or margarine is melted. Whisk in the icing sugar, cocoa powder, and vanilla. It's going to be slightly runny-looking, but that's okay. Cool in the fridge for at least 2 hours. It will be firmer by then. Before icing the cake, beat until fluffy using a hand-held electric mixer. If it's too firm, you can reheat the icing slightly in the microwave or leave it on the counter and then whip with the electric mixer.

10. Now to ice the cake: I love a rustic look when I ice a cake. Place a heaping tablespoon of icing in the centre of a cake stand or plate. Place one of the cake layers on top of it—the icing will help anchor the cake. Divide the icing in half and place one half on top of the first cake layer, spreading it out to the edges. Place the second cake on top of the icing. Spoon on the rest of the icing and evenly spread to the edges. Lastly, lick the bowl because life is too short not to lick the bowl. (Note: There is enough icing to fully ice the cake, albeit it thinly, for anyone who wants a more finished look.)

11. Let the cake set for at least 1 hour and up to 24 hours before slicing. Any leftovers can be stored in an airtight container for up to 2 days.

1 SERVING = 1/16 OF THE CAKE
PER SERVING: 254 CALORIES, 11.5 G TOTAL FAT, 4.7 G SATURATED FAT, 0 G TRANS FAT, 28 MG CHOLESTEROL, 58 MG SODIUM, 44.4 G CARBOHYDRATE, 4.5 G FIBRE, 30.2 G SUGARS, 24.7 G ADDED SUGARS, 2.9 G PROTEIN, 259 MG POTASSIUM
CARBOHYDRATE CHOICE = 3 CHOICES

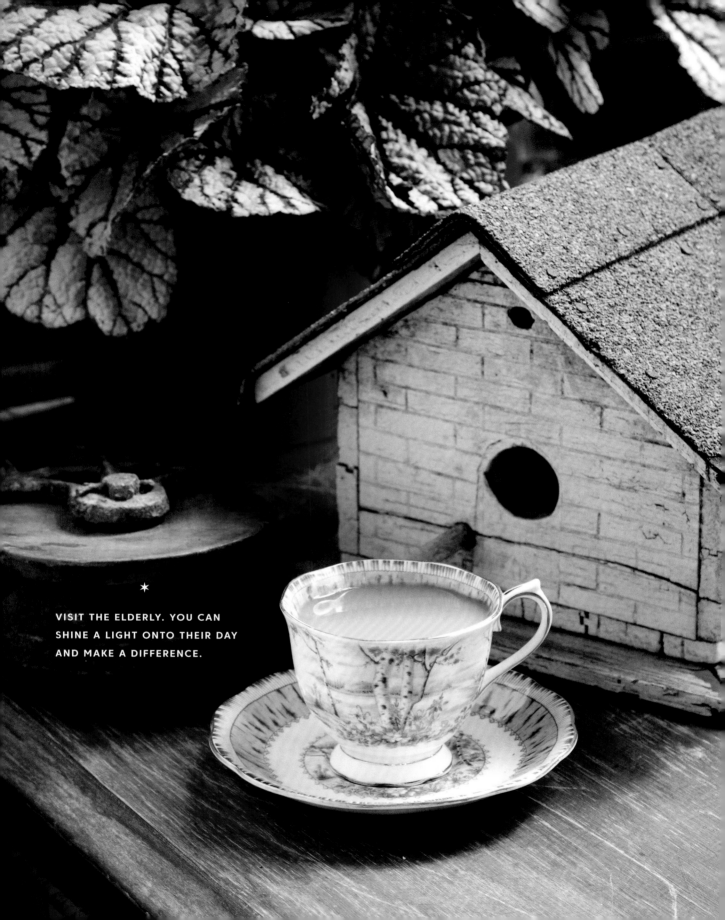

*

VISIT THE ELDERLY. YOU CAN
SHINE A LIGHT ONTO THEIR DAY
AND MAKE A DIFFERENCE.

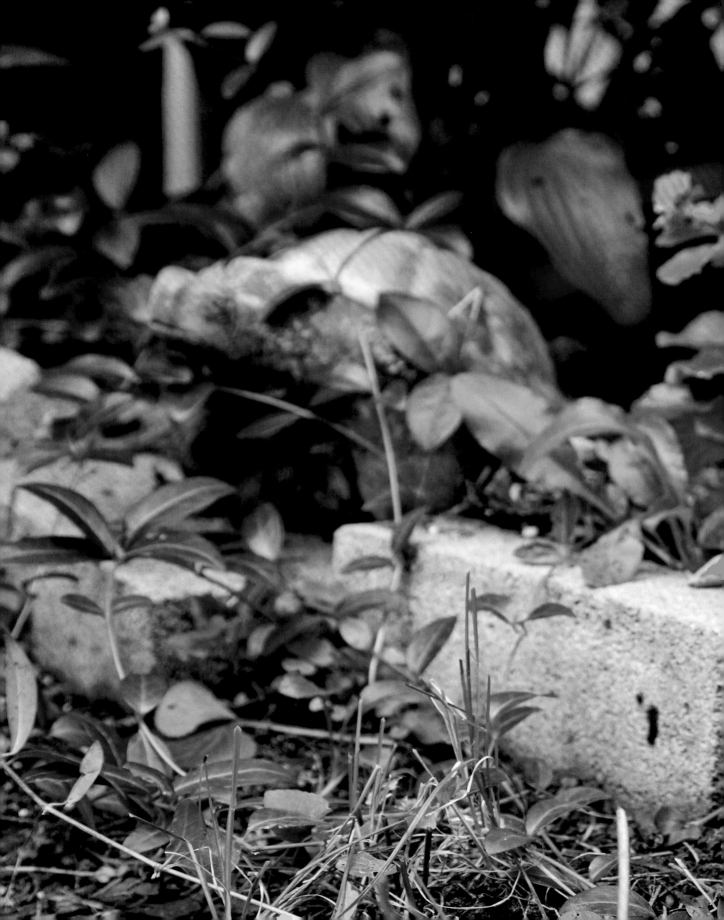

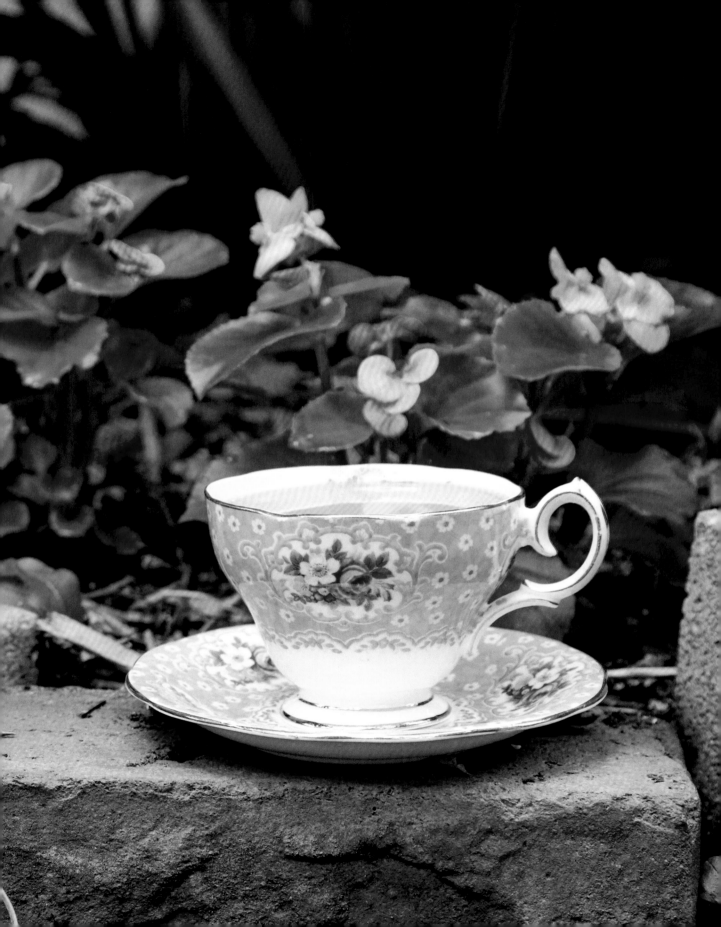

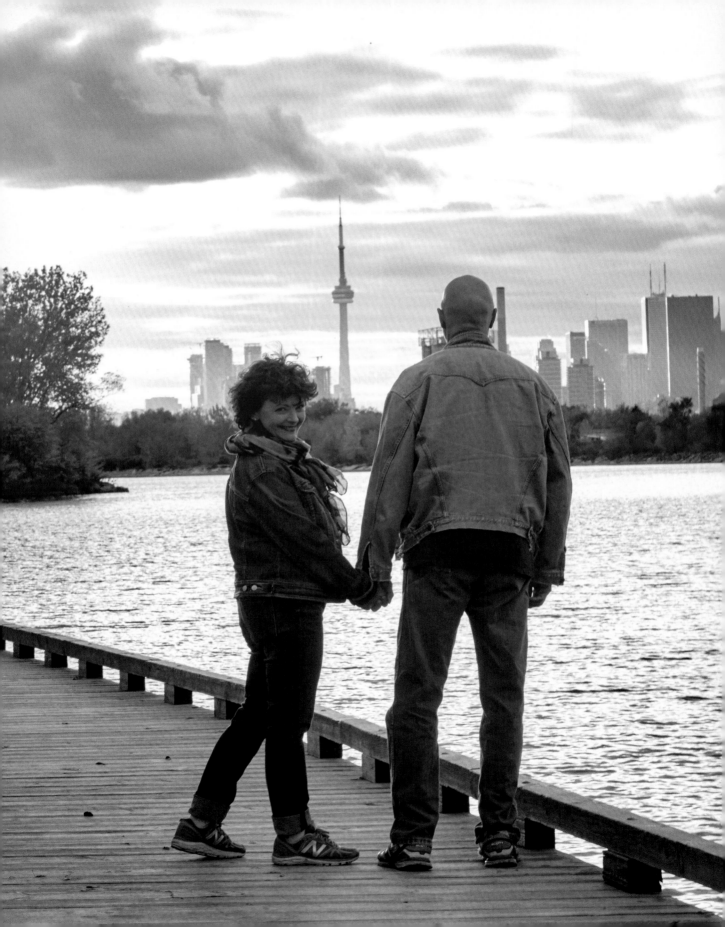

Acknowledgements

EVEN THOUGH MY NAME IS PRINTED ON THE COVER, no one writes a cookbook alone—there are many to thank for their help and support.

First and foremost, I want to thank Robert McCullough, my publisher and friend, for the years of friendship and support and for saying yes to fibre. To my lovely supportive editor and soul sister, Zoe Maslow, who made my writing even better, I have adored working with you from Day 1. A big shout-out to Lisa Jager for her artistic eye. To the entire team at Appetite by Random House, I felt the love the minute I walked through those doors.

I would not have been able to write this cookbook without the love and support of my husband and favourite playmate, Scott. He is my rock.

A huge shout-out and hugs to the members of Team Mairlyn Photo Shoot Days: my favourite photographer, Mike McColl, for his patience, his sense of humour, and the calm energy he brought to a hectic shoot schedule. My fabulous food stylist, Joan Ttooulias, whose eye for detail and wit and laughter kept me going through many a day. My neighbour and food stylist assistant, Erin Spencer, for her enthusiasm and extra props. My BFF, Michale Brode, who tested recipes and single-handedly baked up most of the treats in the treat chapter because I was putting out fires on prep day. My assistant, Katie Brunke, for all her hard work and patience. Tamara Saslove, for helping chop, package, and wash dishes in July. My neighbours, Tom and Evelyne, for letting me use part of their garden during the photo shoot.

My son, Andrew, for trying all my creations and being honest with his comments. And Erin MacGregor, my friend, fellow PHEc and RD, for her fact-checking.

Thank you to my neighbours and recipe testers who tried out my recipes and offered valuable insight: Elise Yanover, Larry Mannell and Jill Harland, Susannah Gray, Faith McGregor, Scott Wickware, Katie Brunke, Mike Tamblyn, Jennifer Dyck, and JC Chessell.

And love to my *Cityline* family, especially the amazing Tracy Moore, and to my *BT Toronto* family, especially the wonderful Dina Pugliese, for their years of support.

Thank you all. Let's party soon.

Index

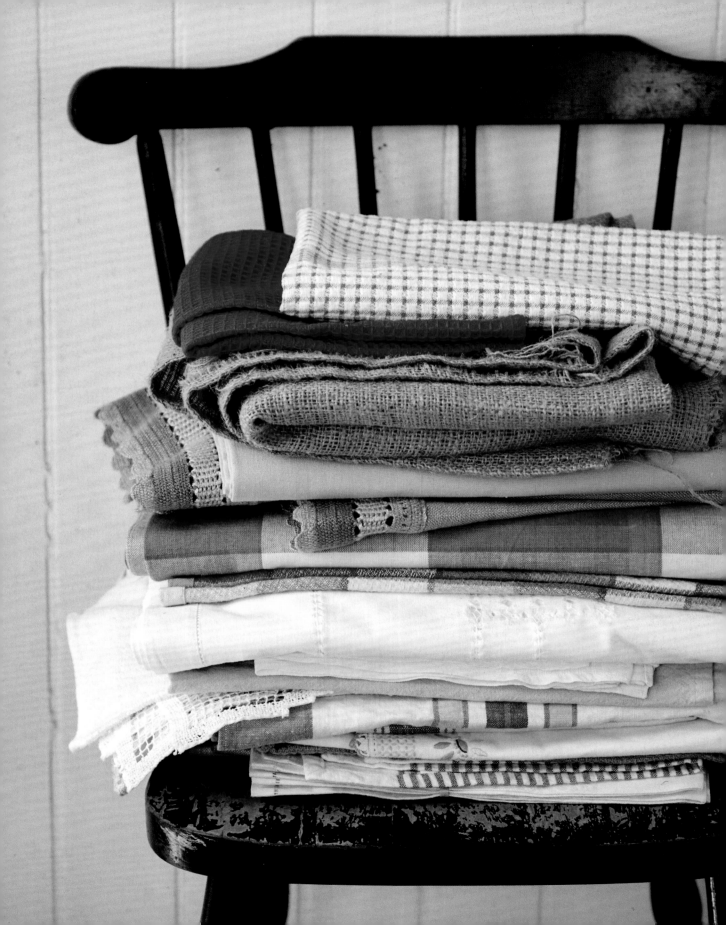